## Praise for *Yoga Through the Ye*

"There is much that we all can learn from trees, nature, and the cycle of the seasons. Aiming to reunite male and female energies, Jilly Shipway brings this inspiration to the practice of yoga. Women are so often excluded from the inner secrets of spiritual practices. Learning to live again in harmony is something wonderful to aspire to."

—Jane Gifford, author of *The Celtic Wisdom of Trees*

"[*Yoga Through the Year*] empowers us to step toward our own authentic holistic wisdom and bring this into our daily yoga practice. Jilly encourages us to align ourselves to our intuitive selves through our inspired personal connection to the seasonal flow of the natural world around us, with mindfulness and gratitude.... Jilly's calm, clear voice shines through this special book, as she guides us though simple, accessible, uncomplicated yoga poses and meditations that connect us to each of the seasons, helping us be more in touch with the earth to deepen our journey with trees and become more aware of our feelings."

—Glennie Kindred, author of *Earth Wisdom*

"*Yoga Through the Year* is a beautiful combination of yoga history and philosophy as well as practices and meditations that invite readers to harmonize with the wisdom of the seasons.... I recommend this book to yoga practitioners of all levels as well as those interested in studying the majesty of the natural world and expanse of the human experience."

—Jennifer Kreatsoulas, PhD, C-IAYT, author of *Body Mindful Yoga*

"This is an inspirational book.... Jilly Shipway steers us safely through an annual spirit-nature trail, with thought-provoking yoga asana practices, meditations, visualizations, creative projects, poetry, and tree wisdom–inspired thoughts.... I thoroughly recommend this book for anyone wishing to explore new territory in their yoga practice throughout the year!"

—Lindy Roy, Viniyoga teacher and Whole Woman Practitioner

"This book encourages the yoga practitioner to tune in to the subtle changes each season brings in. It is enriching to stay open and receptive to the moods and modes each season suggests as it comes into being."

—Sandra Sabatini, author of *Breath: The Essence of Yoga*

"A genuine delight to read. Part yoga guide, part life coach, this book shares in an accessible way some of the key principles of yoga philosophy and marries them with beautiful, flowing yoga practices, sensitive visualizations, and thought-provoking meditation questions. … Jilly is a wise and reassuring presence throughout the book, encouraging us to be present—to this breath, to this moment, to this season—to live and to practice yoga in a way that is respectful of both our bodies and Mother Earth."
—Judy Brenan, British Wheel of Yoga teacher

"*Yoga Through the Year* brilliantly reclaims yoga as a nature-based practice that is perfect for *every* body! Author Jilly Shipway incorporates the wisdom of trees to guide seasonal specific poses, offers personal questions to meditate on, and provides activities designed to internally integrate us into what nature powerfully teaches us throughout the year. … While *Yoga Through the Year* is written for everyone, it is refreshing to finally have a yoga practice that speaks to me: a woman, a witch, and lover of nature!"
—Ruth Barrett, author of *Women's Rites, Women's Mysteries*

"This is a treasure of a book for anyone interested in the seasonal aspects of yoga. Through wisely designed, original, and engaging seasonal practices, Jilly Shipway invites us to listen to and recognize nature's own rhythms within ourselves, and to become healthier and happier human beings in the process."
—Elena Sepúlveda, yoga teacher and editor of *Yogagenda*

"The essence of this book is integration, mind and body, male and female, life and death by using the analogy of the seasons. The techniques of yoga form the primary thread, but mindfulness and compassion and poetry are also woven throughout the narrative. In this age of increasing fragmentation, I can recommend this book as unifying force."
—Professor Janet Treasure, OBE, PhD, award-winning psychiatrist

# YOGA
## THROUGH THE YEAR

## About the Author

Jilly Shipway is a qualified British Wheel of Yoga teacher with more than twenty-five years of teaching experience. Over her long teaching career she has enthused hundreds of students with her love of yoga, and many of them have continued to study with her for many years and up to the present day. She has tutored foundation level, prediploma yoga study courses for the British Wheel of Yoga. She was very fortunate to have discovered yoga in her early teens and so has had a lifetime of studying and practicing yoga. Mindfulness is an integral part of her own yoga practice and her teaching.

As well as teaching general yoga classes, she also has many years of experience teaching specialist yoga classes to adults recovering from mental health problems. She trained at King's College London as a motivational interviewing coach, coaching people caring for someone with an eating disorder, and worked under the supervision of Professor Janet Treasure and her team.

For over ten years Jilly has been developing a seasonal approach to yoga. In tandem with this she has been trying to solve the mystery of women's involvement in the history of yoga. Her Seasonal Yoga courses and website have inspired thousands of yoga practitioners to integrate a seasonal awareness into their yoga practice. She has a BA (Hons) degree in fine art and believes passionately that yoga and mindfulness can really enhance creativity.

Jilly is a regular contributor to the international publication *Yoga Magazine*. When Jilly is not teaching, writing about, or doing yoga, she loves walking in towns, cities, and the wilds of nature. She lives in the UK in a small Welsh border town, surrounded by hills. She is married and has one grown-up daughter.

Visit her website at www.yogathroughtheyear.com.

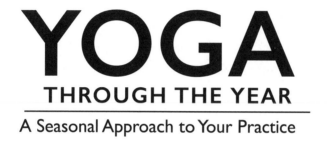

# YOGA
## THROUGH THE YEAR

A Seasonal Approach to Your Practice

JILLY SHIPWAY

Llewellyn Publications
Woodbury, Minnesota

FIRST EDITION
First Printing, 2019

Cover design by Shannon McKuhen
Interior illustrations by Llewellyn Art Department, based on art by Jilly Shipway

Llewellyn is a registered trademark of Llewellyn Worldwide Ltd.

**Library of Congress Cataloging-in-Publication Data**
Names: Shipway, Jilly, author.
Title: Yoga through the year : a seasonal approach to your practice / Jilly
  Shipway.
Description: First Edition. | Woodbury : Llewellyn Worldwide, Ltd., 2019. |
  Includes bibliographical references.
Identifiers: LCCN 2019010088 (print) | LCCN 2019014588 (ebook) | ISBN
  9780738757209 (ebook) | ISBN 9780738756912 (alk. paper)
Subjects: LCSH: Yoga. | Seasons—Miscellanea.
Classification: LCC B132.Y6 (ebook) | LCC B132.Y6 S52135 2019 (print) | DDC
  294.5/436—dc23
LC record available at https://lccn.loc.gov/2019010088

Llewellyn Publications
A Division of Llewellyn Worldwide Ltd.
2143 Wooddale Drive
Woodbury, MN 55125-2989
www.llewellyn.com

Printed in the United States of America

*For my daughter, Kay*

## Disclaimer

Before beginning any new exercise program, it is recommended that you seek medical advice from your healthcare provider. You have full responsibility for your safety and should know your limits. Before practicing asana poses as described in this book, be sure that you are well informed of proper practice and do not take risks beyond your experience and comfort levels. The publisher and the author assume no liability for any injuries caused to the reader that may result from the reader's use of the content contained herein and recommend common sense when contemplating the practices described in the work.

# Contents

# Exercises

## Acknowledgments

Thank you to the earth, the moon, and the sun for giving us the rhythms and the seasons of our lives. You are at the heart of this Seasonal Yoga book.

Thank you to yoga for picking me up when I was a confused, hapless, and ever-hopeful teenager. Thank you for your beauty and diversity and for all the interesting places that you have taken me. Thank you for helping me realize that peace is more than a possibility.

To Glennie Kindred and Ruth Barrett, thank you for all the work that you have both done on the Wheel of the Year, which has given me such a deep well to draw upon.

To Judith Lasater and Donna Farhi, thank you for showing me how to bring my life into yoga and yoga into my life.

Thank you to all the amazing yoga writers, teachers, and practitioners who have helped me expand my definition of what yoga is and what it could be.

I am extremely grateful to Angela Wix, Acquisitions Editor at Llewellyn Publications. I consider Angela to be the midwife to this book! Angela and her team have really helped me pull this book into shape, and I really appreciate all the guidance, help, and support that I have been given by them. Especial thanks to Lauryn Heineman, Lynne Menturweck, Shannon McKuhen, Kat Sanborn, Anna Levine, and Molly McGinnis.

Thank you to all the thousands of peoples who have visited my Seasonal Yoga website, especially those who have contacted me to share their enthusiasm for a seasonal approach to yoga.

I feel very fortunate through my teaching to be able to share my love of yoga, and so a huge thank you to all my students, some of whom have been with me on the path over many years and have taught me so much. Thank you also to local yoga teachers and friends for their friendship and support.

I am very grateful to my group of six readers, who read through my early attempts at chapters for this book and gave me such astute feedback. I really value the expertise, friendship, and support that you have given me, on what at times has been a rocky road. So, thank you to Judy Brenan, Claire Holmes, Lottie Hosie, Linda Poole, Alison Jones, and Ulrike Schade.

Thank you to Rosie Bernard, my niece, for her writerly support and enthusiasm.

To Sue Allen, osteopath, thank you for many years of healing treatments, hand holding, and steadying the ship!

Thank you to my daughter, Kay, for all the joy and happiness you bring into my life. I really appreciate the way that through the whole, long process of writing this book, you have always been there cheering me on!

To Simon, my husband, a big thank you for all that you do and all that you make possible. You bring sunshine into my life through all the seasons.

*Now begins the study and practice of yoga.*

—Yoga Sutra 1:1

# Returning Unity to Yoga
# with the Seasons

If over the millennia yoga had been handed down from mother to daughter through a female lineage, what would an authentic women's yoga be like?

This was the unanswered question that beckoned me onto the path of Seasonal Yoga. Patanjali is considered the father of yoga, and over the millennia yoga has been handed down from father to son, through a male lineage. If Patanjali had had a sister, what is the yoga she would have handed down to us? And if her wisdom had been included in the yoga canon, how would we be different, both on and off our yoga mats? During a period of meditation, I asked (an imaginary) Patanjali's sister for guidance on creating an authentic united yoga. This is the answer that came back to me: "Listen to the earth— that's all. Listen to the earth."

Patanjali's Yoga Sutras are divided into four *padas*, and this gave me the idea to divide my inquiry into one *pada* for each season of the year: spring, summer, autumn, and winter. That is how the seed of Seasonal Yoga was born.

## Understanding the Division of Yoga

My quest to discover a reunited yoga led me to read stories that explained the origins of our male-female division, telling of how women had been spiritually disenfranchised. It appears that Patanjali's sister would have been forbidden to study the sacred texts or to recite mantras, and because she was considered inherently sinful and impure due to her cycles and connection with the earth, she would not have been an appropriate candidate for sacred knowledge.[1]

Because of these things, it is interesting to realize that there is legend of feminine energy within the origins of yoga. I read books that told a fascinating story of how once upon a time God had been considered to be a woman.[2] Hindu scriptures say that the Goddess invented the alphabet and inscribed the first written words onto slabs of stone.[3] That it was women who mapped out the stars and the phases of the moon. That in days gone by her blood had been regarded as holy and her fertility was a cause for celebration and pride. And that both he and she had tended the sacred fire and that the thread of sacred knowledge was held in trust and passed down through the generations, by both him and her. At one time the earth itself was revered as a goddess and the sacred was discovered through our everyday lives on earth.

I also read fascinating tales of the mother origins of yoga. Patanjali is oftentimes referred to as the father of yoga. What is less well known is that Patanjali had a mother and that she was called Gonika.[4] Gonika was a wise woman and she was looking for someone upon whom to bequeath her knowledge of yoga. One day as she stood by a waterfall that flowed into a river, she scooped up a handful of river water into the cupped palms of her hands, and in a worshipful gesture she offered the water to the sun, saying, "This knowledge has come through you; let me give it back to you." Into her praying hands a serpent fell from heaven, and she called him Patanjali. *Pata* means both "serpent" and "fallen"; *anjali* is the worshipful gesture of her cupped hands.

Patanjali did not "father" yoga; rather, he organized the knowledge of yoga that had been handed down to him by his mother, Gonika, into the Yoga Sutras. Legend has it

---

1. Lynn Teskey Denton, *Female Ascetics in Hinduism* (Albany: State University of New York Press, 2004), 25.

2. Merlin Stone, *When God Was a Woman* (Orlando, FL: Harcourt Brace, 1976).

3. Barbara G. Walker, *The Women's Encyclopedia of Myths and Secrets* (New York: HarperCollins Publishers, 1983), 685.

4. B. K. S. Iyengar, *The Tree of Yoga* (London: Thorsons, 2000), 74.

that the yoga that both Patanjali and Gonika inherited was born from the womb of the earth itself. The womb of creation gave birth to the yoga that has been passed down through the generations.[5]

Even though yoga came with this sense of unity, it was lost along the way. Around 200 CE the sage Patanjali compiled the Yoga Sutras, a collection of 196 aphorisms outlining a systematic guide to the practice of yoga. These bite-size chunks of knowledge were passed down orally through the male lineage from father to son.

Patanjali was affiliated with the principles of the classical *Sâmkhya*, a school of thought that proposed that existence consisted of two primordial, interdependent principles: *purusha*, pure consciousness, which is gendered male, and *prakriti*, nature incarnate, which is gendered female. *Purusha* is the observer and *prakriti* is the observed— the seer and the seen. *Prakriti* is the feminine principle, she who gives birth to and creates the manifest world of matter. The aim of yoga, as outlined in Patanjali's Yoga Sutras, is to reach a state of enlightenment by transcending nature. It is a dualistic, transcendent philosophy that outlines the steps required for the yogi to disentangle himself from the natural world and so attain a state of pure consciousness (*samadhi*).

The yoga of Patanjali's Yoga Sutras, known as *Raja Yoga*, the royal path, presents us with a path of transcendence that places the masculine spirit (*purusha*) above feminine matter (*prakriti*). Hence, a schism develops between the natural and the spiritual world. Heaven and earth no longer coexist; they are now on parallel lines destined never to meet. Women are considered to be closer to the earth; they menstruate and give birth and so are considered to be impure; they are also considered to be inherently sinful and so not suited to following the spiritual path. Men are considered to be closer to heaven; they no longer worship the earth; now they worship sky gods. The yoga canon created from this divorce of genders over millennia was devised by a group of people who had never experienced menstruation, pregnancy, giving birth, breastfeeding, or menopause, and so it was only one half of a united experience.

## Reinventing the Wheel of Yoga

Why does it matter what the attitudes toward women were when Patanjali was compiling his Yoga Sutras? Surely today's yoga has moved beyond all this? And yet we are constantly

---

5. Georg Feuerstein, *The Yoga Tradition: Its History, Literature, Philosophy and Practice* (Prescott, AZ: Hohm Press, 2001), 214.

advised to check that the yoga that we practice has an authentic lineage, which will be a male lineage passed down from father to son over millennia.

To create an authentic united yoga we must reunite heaven and earth, and then once again we will rediscover the spiritual within our everyday lives. Spirit no longer transcends the everyday world; rather, it is immanent and found to be within all living things. When women and the earth are rejected as impure and unspiritual, we create a hell on earth. When all genders and the earth are respected and embraced as an important part of spiritual life, we create heaven on earth.

The good news is that we can choose to unite our efforts to a yoga that is healthful, wholesome, and healing. Every time we step onto our yoga mats we can choose to reinvent yoga. With each breath, with each movement, we learn to listen to and love our body and to respect our own and the earth's natural rhythms and cycles. In this way yoga has the potential to be the balm that heals and makes us whole again. Of course, as in acquiring any other skill, it requires practice and discipline. When we reimagine yoga, we all are the richer for it. All genders can then enjoy a yoga that has been made whole again. Heaven and earth are reunited.

## Uniting Yoga with the Ebb and Flow of the Seasons

The word *yoga* can be translated as "union," as in a marriage. This union, or marriage, between complimentary opposites helps us find balance in our lives. *Hatha Yoga* teaches us to look within our self and to discover within our own body the energies of both the sun and the moon. Through our yoga practice we learn to balance our *ha*, solar energy, and our *tha*, lunar energy.

The sun is, quite naturally, at the center of our Seasonal Yoga inquiry. Planet Earth rotates on a tilted axis and revolves around the sun. It is this journey of our planet spinning its way around the sun that gives us the alternating cycles of night and day, light and dark, summer and winter.

Modern-day life in the twenty-first century is fast-paced and unrelenting. We can be turned on and tuned in twenty-four hours a day. Our 24/7 society means that many of us work longer and more unsociable hours, which can take a heavy toll on body, mind, and soul. The boundaries between public space and private space have become blurred; and so, it can be more difficult to withdraw and simply take time out just to be. We recognize that there are many benefits to modern-day living, but our health is endangered when we disconnect from our own and the earth's natural rhythms. When we marry seasonal awareness with our yoga practice, a path that leads to a saner, healthier, more balanced, and more harmonious way of living is revealed to us.

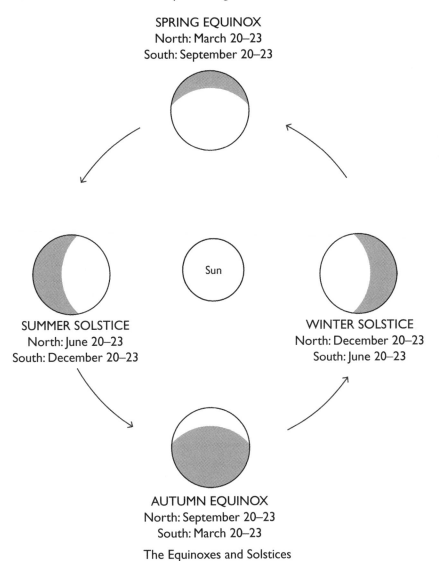

**SPRING EQUINOX**
North: March 20–23
South: September 20–23

**SUMMER SOLSTICE**
North: June 20–23
South: December 20–23

Sun

**WINTER SOLSTICE**
North: December 20–23
South: June 20–23

**AUTUMN EQUINOX**
North: September 20–23
South: March 20–23

The Equinoxes and Solstices

There is an ebb and flow to our lives: the sun rises, the sun sets; tides rise and fall; the moon waxes and wanes. A flower, our heart, the moon, the sea—all these things have a rhythm. A flower opens and closes its petals in response to dawn and dusk. The year ebbs and flows in a perpetual dance of sunlight and shadow. Like the moon, the year also has periods of waxing and waning. An awareness of this ebb and flow of the year can help us know when it is a good time to push forward and take action and when it is better to take a more contemplative approach. It also helps us feel connected to and supported by the earth.

On the one hand, our yoga practice takes us on a journey inward that leads us along a path that spirals into the very center of our being, and the prize is self-knowledge. On the other hand, when we develop an awareness of, and a connection to, the seasons, we are led along a path that spirals outward and leads us to attaining knowledge of the world and beyond. Our yoga practice reveals to us a cosmos within ourselves that is a mirror image of the outer cosmos. Our seasonal awareness connects us to the outer world as it is in the here and now. With dedicated and sincere practice of both yoga and seasonal awareness, we gain an enlightened realization of the nature of our true selves and of the world.

One of the simplest ways of developing a seasonal awareness is to become aware of and to observe the four cardinal solar points around the wheel of the year. These are the two solstices and the two equinoxes.

- The winter solstice is when we have the shortest day.
- The summer solstice is when we have the longest day.
- The spring equinox is when day and night are of equal length before we tip into the lightest phase of the year.
- The autumn equinox is when day and night are of equal length before we tip into the darkest phase of the year.

Broadly speaking, for our Seasonal Yoga inquiry we can divide the year into two halves. Between the winter solstice and the summer solstice is the "light" half of the year, when the days are getting longer. Between the summer solstice and the winter solstice is the "dark" half of the year, when the nights are getting longer. Your first steps on the path of Seasonal Yoga might be to simply work with the wheel of the year to develop an awareness of where you are energy-wise in the year. You can then pinpoint whether you are in the lighter or darker half of the year and whether the sun's energy is waxing or waning.

The light half of the year, between the winter solstice and the summer solstice, can be compared to the inhalation. It is energizing, is expansive, and supports activity. It is associated with sunlight, fire, radiating, expansion, waxing, pushing, effort, action, extroversion, and outer activities.

The light half of the year takes us from the heart of winter to the height of summer. During this time, the sun's energy is waxing, the light is expanding, and the days are getting longer and warmer. We move from winter into spring and then into summer. This is the growing season, and seeds that are planted now will grow and expand. Generally speaking, this light half of the year favors an outward focus, with an emphasis on action and outward achievements. We use the season's fiery, expansive energy to make things happen and to get things done. During the light half of the year, our yoga practice can help us stay connected to our inner wisdom and be guided by it when taking action in the world.

The dark half of the year between the summer solstice and the winter solstice can be compared to the exhalation. It is relaxing, regenerating, renewing and supports letting go. It is associated with moon, night, waning, drawing inward, yielding, incubation, hibernation, reflection, contemplation, rest, and regeneration.

The dark half of the year takes us from the height of summer into the depths of winter. During this time, the sun's energy is waning, the dark is expanding, and the days are getting shorter and nights longer. We move from summer to autumn and into winter. As autumn and winter progress, nature starts to gradually die back, and we enter a period of dormancy and decay. Broadly speaking, the dark half of the year favors an inward focus, with an emphasis on contemplation and rest. We use the watery energy of the season to incubate ideas, to find rest and renewal, and to dream and plan. During the dark half of the year, our yoga practice can help us remain positive and stay connected to our inner light.

As we gain more experience working with the wheel of the year, we learn to recognize and work with the season's alternating cycles of light and dark, and to more skillfully ride the prevailing energy of the season. The common thread that runs through both our yoga practice, and our work with the seasons, is that both disciplines teach us the wisdom of when it is better to push and when it is better to yield.

In his Yoga Sutras Patanjali has very little to say about the practice of *asana*, other than in Yoga Sutra 2:46: *Sthira-sukham asanam,* or "Asana must have the dual quality of alertness and relaxation."[6] In other words, we maintain a state of equanimity in a challenging yoga pose by learning to balance pushing and yielding. In yoga this is referred to as balancing effort (*sthira*) with relaxation (*sukha*). The word *sthira* can be translated as steadiness, firmness, alertness, strength, or effort. The word *sukha* can be translated as comfort, agreeable, flexible, or relaxation.

As you become more experienced at recognizing the prevalent pushing or yielding energy of the season, you will also fine-tune your ability to choose yoga practices that balance your own energy flow. For example, in winter there is a natural tendency to want to hibernate, so you might honor this by choosing restful, restorative (*langhana*) poses. On the other hand, in winter you might also want to choose energizing (*brahmana*) poses to boost your happy hormones and ward off the winter blues.

When practicing yoga, the breath provides a perfect barometer to measure whether we have achieved the correct balance between effort and relaxation. Our yoga practice teaches us to ride the ebb and flow of the breath, which in turn prepares us to skillfully ride the ebb and flow of the seasons in an ever-changing world. We learn to befriend and observe the breath, and the quality of the breath gives us clues to whether we are putting in too much or too little effort. If the breathing becomes ragged, labored, or erratic we know that our practice has become too effortful and we need to balance this with a more relaxed approach. We are aiming for a long, smooth, even, calming breathing pattern.

The beauty of the Seasonal Yoga approach is that it is tailor-made to fit your needs during every season of the year. Each of the seasonal chapters in this book will help you familiarize yourself with the prevalent energy of the season and show you how you can use this awareness to create balance in both your yoga practice and your life.

## How to Use This Book

You can dip into this book all year round to find seasonal inspiration and guidance. Each of the eight seasonal chapters consists of the following elements:

---

6. T. K. V. Desikachar, *The Heart of Yoga: Developing Personal Practice* (Rochester, VT: Inner Traditions International, 1995), 180.

- Summary of the relevant seasonal themes and pointers for how best to work with the opportunities and challenges of the season
- Yoga practice inspired by the season
- Seasonal meditation or visualization
- Tree wisdom section
- Set of seasonal meditation questions

Although most of the elements of the book are self-explanatory, to get the full benefit of the book, I recommend that all readers start by reading chapter 1. After that, you could either read through the whole book, which will give you a feel for the Seasonal Yoga approach, or dip into the book season by season to get ideas for the season you are in.

The various mindfulness exercises, visualizations, meditations, and yoga practices in this book have all been chosen to be specifically relevant for a particular season. However, if you like a particular practice, it's fine to use it throughout the year.

I hope that this book is one that you will return to often over the seasons and across the years. Each time you use the methods outlined in the book you will increase your confidence to tune in to and align yourself with the seasonal energy, and you will gradually, over time and with experience, establish your own rhythm of responding to the changing seasons. I hope that the outcome of this is that you learn to care for yourself, your loved ones, and the planet in a sustainable, loving, and compassionate way.

# CHAPTER ONE

# The Seasonal Yoga Practice

This chapter gives you guidance on how to work with the key seasonal practices described in the book, which include Seasonal Yoga asana practices, the Seasonal Yoga meditation questions, and tree wisdom practices. You will get the most out of the book if you read through this chapter first, and it will build your confidence in your ability to use the Seasonal Yoga practices. Once you have read this chapter, you are ready to confidently dive into the seasonal chapters that follow.

## Seasonal Yoga Asana Practices

Each of the seasonal chapters has its own Seasonal Yoga asana practice, and these practices will give you a way of keeping fit, flexible, calm, and energized all year round. They will allow you to connect with the rhythm of the year and align your energy to that rhythm, promoting happiness, health, and harmony in every season.

There are eight Seasonal Yoga practices, one for each of the four cardinal points around the wheel of the year (the winter and summer solstices and the spring and autumn equinoxes) and one for each of the four seasonal transition points (e.g., winter to spring). The eight Seasonal Yoga practices will provide you with a tailor-made year-round set of yoga routines.

All the yoga practices have been designed to be appropriate for a specific season; however, if you particularly like one of the practices, it's fine to use it all year round.

Many of us lead busy lives, and so the yoga practices in this book have been designed to be a manageable length that will easily fit into your daily life. Each practice takes between ten and thirty minutes, so even on the busiest of days you'll probably be able to fit in some yoga. By doing some yoga, you'll end up feeling calmer and less time-pressured.

The Seasonal Yoga approach is for everybody. All the practices are easy to follow and accessible. You don't need to be super fit or hyper-flexible to do these yoga routines. You won't be asked to tie yourself in knots or to get into impossible pretzel-like positions (although if pretzel-like yoga poses are your thing, there is no reason why you shouldn't adapt the Seasonal Yoga approach to encompass this way of working).

The English and Sanskrit (an ancient Indo-European language of India) names are given for each of the yoga poses (*asanas*) used in the book. If you want more information about a yoga pose, it's easy to find with a quick internet search using the pose name. If you are new to yoga and unfamiliar with the poses described, think about attending a class to allow you to learn the positions correctly. See also the recommended resources section at the end of this book.

The eight Seasonal Yoga practices can act as a springboard for creating your own Seasonal Yoga practices. If you are a follower of a particular type of yoga, I encourage you to integrate some of the Seasonal Yoga ideas into your own form of yoga.

Simple, uncomplicated, accessible yoga poses and routines have been chosen so that they can be approached in a mindful, meditative way. The emphasis is not on achieving gymnastic-type poses; rather, it's on being present to the breath, moment by moment, for the duration of the practice. Guidance has been given on coordinating the breath with the movements, which supports this meditative approach. Never strain with the breathing. If you are new to yoga, while you are learning the poses, you might prefer just to let the breath take care of itself.

Mindfulness practitioners could use the eight Seasonal Yoga practices in this book as the mindful movement component of their regular mindfulness practice.

## Seasonal Meditation Questions

The seasonal meditation questions are a key component of the Seasonal Yoga approach, and each of the eight seasonal chapters in this book concludes with a set of meditation questions. We use them every six weeks or so to correspond with the solstices, equinoxes, and seasonal transition points (each chapter will give you dates for working with the questions). The questions are a series of open inquiries that will help you do the following:

- Connect with the season you are in.
- Reflect on how you wish to use your energy and set your intentions for the coming season.
- Look back over the previous season, celebrating your successes and learning from the seeds that failed to germinate.
- Know when the best time is to plant seeds of intention, giving them the best chance of growing and blossoming.
- Learn how to align your own energy with the prevalent energy of the season and know which time favors contemplation or action. Use your knowledge of the seasonal energy to balance periods of activity and rest.
- The meditation questions combined with a meditative approach will give you access to the deep wisdom of your subconscious mind.

By working with the meditation questions, you can become your own year-round life coach. Each set of questions encourages you to review all aspects of your life, including relationships, work (or study/home management), self-care, and community or environmental involvement. The questions help you get a good work-life balance by encouraging you to give attention to all aspects of your life, rather than getting over-focused on one particular area. By stopping every six weeks or so to use the meditation questions, you have a chance to review progress in all areas of your life, and if you have gone off track, you have the chance to correct yourself and get back on course again. I find using the meditation questions helps me to realize who and what are important to me and to direct my energy accordingly.

Here is an example of some meditation questions that are designed to be used around the time of Spring Equinox. These questions are on the theme of how you wish to channel your energy work-wise during the coming season.

- During the growing season, whatever we unite our energy with will expand and grow. How will I make best use of the fertile energy of the coming growing season?
  - ↪ Which projects do I wish to prioritize?
  - ↪ What lights my fire and what am I passionate about?
  - ↪ What actions will I need to take to ensure that the projects most dear to my heart come to fruition?
  - ↪ What should I say no to in order to create the space to say yes to the things that really matter to me? (What needs to be cut back or pruned?)
  - ↪ Who are my allies? Who can I enlist support from? Who shares my vision and will help me to make my dreams become a reality?

The meditation questions for each season have been devised in such a way that you can either devote a lot of time to them or very little. For those of you who are short of time, there are a few quick and easy ways of working with the questions. Simply read the meditation questions through before you go to bed and trust that your subconscious and universal conscious will come up with answers to the questions. You might also integrate one of the questions into an activity that you are doing anyway, such as walking to your car, walking along a corridor at work, exercising at the gym, jogging, showering, and so on.

If you have 10 to 30 minutes available, then the seasonal meditation questions can be used in yoga sessions, sitting meditations, writing meditations, informal walking meditations, and formal walking meditations. I'll discuss each of these five options in more details next.

## Integrating Seasonal Meditation Questions into Your Yoga Practice

Our yoga practice provides us with a brilliant way of accessing the subconscious mind. Seasonal Yoga meditation questions can be integrated into a yoga session in several ways:

- You can include a meditation question during either a sitting meditation or a period of yoga relaxation, either at the beginning or end of your yoga practice.
- You can turn a meditation question over in your mind as you hold a resting pose, such as the Mountain Pose (*Tadasana*), Easy Pose (*Sukhasana*), or Child Pose (*Balasana*).
- You can hold a meditation question in your mind as you stay and hold a yoga pose for a few breaths.

During your yoga practice, all you need to do is to pose a meditation question and then let it go, trusting that your subconscious mind will at some point come up with an answer to the question.

EXERCISE

## Sitting Meditation

The Seasonal Yoga meditation questions can be used during a period of sitting meditation to calm and focus the mind.

The sitting meditation with meditation questions can be done anywhere and anytime.

It can be done either as a formal sitting meditation on your own in a safe space or less formally, by, for example, taking a few minutes as a break from the computer or during your commute to work (by public transport only—do not meditate when you are driving!). Remember to set a timer, if that's your preference.

Find yourself a comfortable but erect sitting position, either in a straight-backed, upright chair or on the floor (if sitting is difficult, this meditation can be done lying down). Notice where your body is in contact with the floor or your support and the sensations associated with this. Become aware of the natural flow of your breath. Throughout the meditation keep a gentle, background awareness of the flow of your breath and any bodily sensations.

Choose one of the meditation questions and begin to turn it over in your mind. Hold the question lightly. If your mind wanders off, gently bring it back to an awareness of your body, your breathing, and the meditation question.

Notice any ideas that come into your head in response to the question. Allow yourself the freedom to explore these ideas and see where they take you. Be gently vigilant, and if your attention is hijacked by everyday preoccupations or worries, gently but firmly bring your awareness back to the meditation question that you have chosen to focus on. Enjoy exploring the ideas that surface in response to this question.

When you feel ready (and if you have time), choose another question to meditate upon.

End the meditation by sitting quietly for a few breaths; notice where your body is in contact with the floor or your support; become aware of your surroundings. You might want to jot down any ideas or insights that have come to you during your sitting meditation. Or, if you have time, follow this sitting meditation with a writing meditation.

EXERCISE
## Writing Meditation

The writing meditation can be done as a stand-alone meditation, can follow the sitting or walking meditations, or can come before or after your yoga practice.

Combining a writing meditation with meditation questions is an effective way to get your ideas flowing and gain access to the wisdom of your subconscious mind. If your creativity is blocked, this meditation will fire up your imagination. If you have come to an impasse in your life, it will help you reorient and get you moving forward again.

Personally, I like the physicality of writing with pen and paper. However, it's fine to work digitally too. Either way, have your writing materials in hand.

Choose a meditation question. Set your timer for 10 to 20 minutes and start writing. Keep your pen in contact with the paper and keep writing until your timer goes.

Write down whatever comes into your head in response to the meditation questions. Your aim is to capture the stream of thoughts and feelings as they flow through your mind. Let go of your inner editor! It doesn't matter how off the wall your thoughts are—just get them down! Later, after the meditation has finished, you can read through and separate the nuggets of gold from the stones and grit. But for now just keep that pen moving!

Be reassured that whatever you write down during your meditation is for your eyes only. No need to pay attention to handwriting, neatness, spelling, grammar, presentation, and so on. As long as your writing is legible and comprehensible to you, anything goes.

Be aware of the physical act of writing and how it feels to be someone sitting here writing. Relax any parts of your body that do not need to be engaged with the act of writing. If you find that you are tensing up, slow your writing down, consciously relax, and reconnect with the flow of your breath. At the same time, keep writing! A relaxed attitude will help you to access your subconscious mind, and it is here that we uncover our gold.

However, it's no problem if you find it impossible to relax—just keep on writing anyway. Part of your meditation can be to write, and at the same time maintain a gentle awareness of how it feels to be tense, noticing sensations as they arise in your body. If you can't let it go, then just let it be.

Once your timer goes, put your pen down, notice how your body feels, how you are feeling in yourself, and the natural flow of your breath. Be aware of where your body is in contact with the floor or your chair. And when you are ready, carry on with your day.

At the end of the writing meditation you might want immediately to read what you have written or you might prefer to look over it later. It's a good idea to keep your writing, and then over several years of practice, you will see how the seasons of your life have changed as well as the seasons of the year.

<hr>

### EXERCISE
# Informal Walking Meditation

An informal walking meditation, combined with meditation questions, can easily be fitted into your day without any need to find extra time. It's a way of getting gentle exercise and it's relaxing as well. Walking clears your mind and helps ideas flow better. Being outside in the open air helps you feel connected to nature and the seasons.

This walking meditation can be done either indoors or out, any time that you have to walk somewhere. It can be done in your house, in your office, or while walking from your car to home or workplace. It can be done in the city, the country, a park, or a shopping mall. Do remember to stay safe and be aware of any hazards as you walk.

Take enjoyment in the act of walking and your surroundings: the sights, sounds, and aromas. Notice how it feels to be walking, especially the contact between your feet and the earth beneath you. Maintain a gentle awareness of your natural breathing as you walk.

When you are ready, begin to turn one of the meditation questions over in your mind as you walk. Hold the question lightly; you don't need to try too hard to find an answer to the question. Just trust that at some point your subconscious mind will come up with an answer. If your mind wanders off, gently bring it back to an awareness of your surroundings, your body, your breathing, and the meditation question.

Notice any ideas that come into your head in response to the question. Feel free to explore these ideas and see where they lead you. Be gently vigilant, and if you notice your attention getting hijacked by everyday preoccupations, concerns, and worries, just gently but firmly bring it back to the question. Enjoy exploring any ideas that surface in response to the question.

When you feel ready (and if you have time), choose another question to meditate upon.

At the end of your walk, you might want to jot down any inspiration, ideas, or insights that surfaced during your meditation. Or if you have time, follow this informal walking meditation with a writing meditation.

## EXERCISE
# Formal Walking Meditation

A formal walking meditation is walking meditatively on a specific circuit for a specified amount of time.

A formal walking meditation combined with meditation questions is relaxing and a way of getting gentle exercise. Walking clears the mind and helps ideas flow. It has a grounding and centering effect. For the reluctant meditator it can be an enjoyable way into meditation.

First decide where you are going to walk. Your walking circuit could be inside or outside and could involve walking from one side of a room to the other and back again or walking in a circle. Choose somewhere you feel safe and will not be disturbed, such as a room in your house, a hallway, your garden, a local park, an unused room at your gym, or a corridor at work.

It's a good idea to set a timer and commit to walking for a specific amount of time. Ten minutes is ideal, but you can do more if you wish.

Start the meditation by becoming aware of how it feels to walk, noticing the contact between your feet and the earth and any sensations you feel in the feet. Keep a background awareness of how your whole body feels as you walk. Maintain a gentle awareness of the natural flow of your breath. Take enjoyment from the act of walking.

Begin to turn a meditation question over in your head as you walk. Hold the question lightly. If your mind wanders off, gently bring it back to an awareness of your body walking, your breathing, and the meditation question. Notice any ideas that come into your head in response to the question. Allow yourself the freedom to explore these ideas and see where they lead you. Be gently vigilant, and if your attention is hijacked by everyday preoccupations or worries, gently but firmly bring it back to the question that you are focusing on. When you feel ready (and if you have time), choose another question to meditate upon.

When your timer goes, at the end of your walking meditation, you might want to jot down any ideas, inspiration, or insights that came to you. Or, if you have time, follow this formal walking meditation with a writing meditation.

———

The seasonal meditation questions are an accessible way to begin your Seasonal Yoga journey. And if you commit to devoting some time to working with them every six weeks or so, your life will be enriched for it. Once you are in the habit of using them regularly, your life flows better, you're well positioned to take advantage of opportunities that come your way, and you'll find ways to make your dreams come true!

## Tree Wisdom as a Guide through Our Seasonal Yoga Practice

In addition to the Seasonal Yoga practices and meditation questions, each of the seasonal chapters contains a tree wisdom section. This will help you connect to the seasons and enhance your creativity.

Yoga is union and trees are a living, breathing embodiment of this union. The tree embodies all of yoga's teachings, and so trees make a wonderful guru. The aim of yoga is to create a state of balanced perfection by uniting complimentary opposites in a harmonious union. The tree marries earth to sky and stands perfectly balanced between the two. A tree is Mother Earth made visible and tangible to us. Touch any leaf on any tree and you are touching our star, the sun. Trees are the earth's lungs, breathing in carbon dioxide and breathing out oxygen. No matter who you are, where you are, or what you are like, trees breathe life into you. Is it any coincidence that the Buddha found enlightenment under a tree?

Where tree meets sky is the spaciousness of yoga. Where tree connects with earth is the groundedness of yoga. Where tree stands in space is the peaceful centeredness of yoga. The tree stands at the center of its own circle, and daily life rotates around it. Even within the frantic rush of city life we can always find a moment of peace when we rest our gaze upon a tree.

Trees connect us to the changing seasons and to life itself. When we connect with trees, we connect with earth, air, fire, and water. Spending time around them is healing and they help us recover from illness and reduce our stress levels. They filter our air and reduce pollution, cool our cities, and purify our water. They bring the seasons into the city and remind us that our home is both earth and sky.

I have always felt a connection to trees. My mum is of a generation of people who were instructed by the baby experts of the time to leave their baby outside in the fresh air; consequently, when I was a baby, I spent many hours parked under a tree in my pram. Inside the house my mum would be doing her chores, and outside in the garden I would be staring in baby wonder up at the treetops gently blowing in the breeze. Even now when I am in a state of deep meditation, my awareness will oftentimes fly off to the top of trees and float unfettered in baby-like bliss there.

In our relationship with trees we humans act as though we are the superior partner. We throw our weight around, clearing forests and polluting the earth, water, and air. Trees clean up after us, filtering our air, purifying our water, and mopping up the pollution that we've created. In truth it is not an equal relationship because in reality we need trees far more than they need us. Trees inspire us with life: they breathe in carbon dioxide and breathe out oxygen, and we breathe in oxygen and breathe out carbon dioxide. Our breath connects us to trees.

In India trees are venerated as *vanas devatas* (forest deities). Women in rural India have played a significant part in protesting against the cutting of trees. In Rajasthan about three hundred years ago the followers of a Hindu sect called *Bishnoi*, led by a woman called Amrita Devi, protected the trees by embracing them and so shielding them from being felled by the woodcutters. Imagine loving trees so much that you are prepared to put your own body in harm's way to protect them from harm. *Ahimsa* (non-violence or non-harm) is a cardinal principle of yoga philosophy. When we abuse nature, we abuse ourselves. When we love and treat nature with respect, we love and treat ourselves with respect.

Over the past year, while I have been writing this book, I have been on a tree pilgrimage. On this pilgrimage I have visited valleys, wildflower meadows, woodlands, cornfields, gardens, city sidewalks, churchyards, mountains, hillsides, and wild moorlands. From this experience I have been inspired to compose seasonal tree meditation poems that will help you connect on a deep spiritual, emotional, and physical level with trees. The tree meditation poems can be used in many ways: for example, you could read one of the poems at the start of your yoga practice and let it to do its tree magic and inspire your yoga session. Or if you are a yoga teacher, you could read it to your class at the start of a period of relaxation or meditation.

Each tree has taught me a valuable lesson and given me a gift, which is reflected in the meditation poem I have written about it:

- The **willow tree** has taught me to listen to the wind whispering that spring is here.

- The **apple tree** has taught me how to stay effortlessly in touch with that which is light, pure, beautiful, and graceful within me and how it is possible to blossom in a world that is neither perfect nor pure.

- The **oak tree** has taught me about the strength and generosity contained within the circle of life, death, rebirth, and renewal.

- The **crab apple tree** has taught me that contained within the ordinary, everyday world, there is concealed a secret, magical, beautiful core that is ripe with potential and possibility.

- The **sycamore tree** has taught me to simply *be* in the midst of all the *doing* and to stay at the center of the circle and let all things take their course.

- The **yew tree** has taught me to look for the sacred and holy within nature and that healing will naturally follow.

- The **holly tree** has taught me to dance through the seasons and to stay connected to my joy even on the darkest and coldest of winter days.

- The **rowan tree** has taught me how to create an extraordinary, magical gift out of ordinary, everyday ingredients and to keep on giving that gift the whole year round.

Along with the tree meditation poem, you will also find additional information and activities in the Tree Wisdom sections. These will give you inspiration and ideas on how to develop both mindfulness and creativity by spending time around trees.

EXERCISE

## Standing Like a Tree

This exercise can be used at any time of year as a stand-alone exercise or as part of your yoga practice. It can be used as a way of centering and grounding yourself at the start of a yoga practice. In daily life it is particularly helpful for those times when you feel thrown off balance by a situation and need to regain your equilibrium and ground yourself.

Stand tall like a tree. Your feet are parallel and about hip width apart. Your knees are soft, your face relaxed, shoulders down away from the ears. Your tailbone feels heavy as though it is weighted, and the crown of your head feels light and floats skyward. Picture in your mind's eye a tree that you love or feel a connection to.

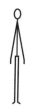

Standing Like a Tree

Bring your awareness to your feet. Be aware of where your feet are in contact with the earth beneath you. Allow your toes to spread and your heels to drop down into the earth. Imagine that there are roots growing from the soles of your feet, going deep down into the earth below you, spreading in a wide circle, and giving you stability.

With each inhale imagine that you are drawing healing energy and nourishment up though your roots into the soles of your feet, up through the legs, torso, and lungs.

With each exhale imagine that the out-breath is traveling down both legs, through your feet, and back down into your roots. Imagine with each exhale that you are letting go of anything that you do not wish to hold on to, letting go of tension, worries, anxiety, persistent thoughts, discomfort, or pain. Imagine that any negativity that you let go of is then cleansed and purified by the soil.

**Inhale:** Healing energy

**Exhale:** Letting go

Repeat over several breaths until you feel centered and grounded.

———

Now that you are familiar with how to use the different Seasonal Yoga practices, you could either read through the whole of the book (this will give you a feel for the Seasonal Yoga approach) or dip into the book chapter by chapter to get ideas for the season you are in.

# CHAPTER TWO

# Spring Equinox

*March 20–23 in the Northern Hemisphere*
*September 20–23 in the Southern Hemisphere*

The spring equinox is a good time to consider how we go about creating a balanced life. Yoga is a union, a marriage between complementary opposites that helps us find balance in our lives.

## The Sun Is Rising in the Heavens

In ancient times the beginning of the year was reckoned from this moment, at the spring equinox, when the sun crossed the equator and began rising higher each day in the heavens.

The spring equinox is a solar festival celebrated when the length of day and night are equal. The word *equinox* comes from Latin and means "equal night." In our yoga practice we can explore the equinox theme of balance by working with yoga's balancing poses. We can also reflect on how best to balance our own sun (*ha*) and moon (*tha*) energies, both in our yoga practice and in our life. Yoga helps us reconcile opposing parts of our self, creating optimum conditions for healing to occur.

The spring equinox is the ignition key for the year, and from here the energy of the year really revs up. There is a short-lived period of fertile energy during the growing season as the days get longer and warmer between now and the summer solstice. In days gone by, Eostre, the earth goddess of fertility and new life, was honored at this time. Her name is the root of the word we give to the female hormone *estrogen*. The tradition of the Easter Bunny and the giving of chocolate eggs at Easter are all connected to the celebration of fertility at the equinox.

Whatever seeds are planted now will expand and grow. At this time we have an outward focus, and our face is turned toward the sun. This is a time for pushing rather than for yielding. We need to prioritize and use this short-lived, fertile sun energy to grow and make manifest the projects that are closest to our heart. Our actions will be more effective and successful if we have strategies in place. We look for opportunities to reach out to others, make connections, and collaborate with those people who will help us realize our dreams.

Our yoga practice can help us stay in touch with our inner wisdom as we take action in the world. In this way we can take wise actions that come from the heart. We can also use our yoga practice to stay balanced, centered, and grounded so that we are not swept away by the restless, frantic energy of the growing season.

## Finding Balance at the Spring Equinox

The spring equinox is a good time to consider how we go about creating a balanced life. Our yoga practice teaches us to balance tension and relaxation. Our challenge is, how do we marry and unify these two complimentary opposites to achieve a state of balance in our lives?

In the opening words of the Yoga Sutras Patanjali defines yoga as the cessation of the turning of thoughts in the mind. Many of us are drawn to yoga initially hoping that it will help still our restless, agitated mind. With the changes and surge in energy that spring brings, some of us find our mind speeds up too, which can leave us feeling unbalanced, anxious, and overwhelmed. Later in this chapter you will find practices, such as the Calming Cloud Meditation, to help restore your equilibrium in the face of this onslaught of airy, adrenalized spring-time energy.

As yoga practitioners, we can learn the art of balance by observing the earth's graceful seasonal transition in and out of balanced states at the equinoxes. At both equinoxes the earth is temporarily balanced between light and dark, night and day, before it tips either into the lighter or darker half of the year. At the autumn equinox the earth is in a balanced state before it tips into the dark, dormant (*tamas*) phase of the year when everything dies back. At the spring equinox there is balance before we tip into the light, active (*rajas*) growing season phase of the year. When we observe the seasonal changes, we see that there is a seasonal cycle of balance, activity, balance, and rest; and then the cycle begins again.

We may wrongly get the impression from the yoga media that yoga is about creating a stress-free, blissful life. Seductive images of the young and beautiful practicing yoga on sun-drenched, paradise island beaches might contrast sharply with our own sometimes messy and chaotic life. However, when we conceive of yoga as perfect peace that is only to be found on some faraway island, a profound mismatch develops between our life as it is in the here and now and our life as we would like it to be. On the one hand, this discrepancy may lead us to make changes in our life that make it more harmonious and peaceful. On the other hand, it may lead to a profound dissatisfaction and a sense that neither we nor our lives are quite good enough to match up to yoga's ideals.

Our yoga practice can introduce an element of tension into our lives if we strive to be in a state of perpetual yogic relaxation. When we struggle to be our best yogic self at all times, a battle ensues between the so-called yogic and non-yogic parts of ourselves. In an attempt to create a bubble of yoga serenity, we push away all that threatens to burst that bubble. We stop listening to the news and avoid situations that bring up difficult feelings such as anxiety, and when "negative" emotions such as anger arise, we put a yogic half-smile on our face and attempt to keep calm and carry on!

How do we reconcile the inevitable tension that arises in life with our wish to be relaxed and calm? We can return to the example set for us by Earth on its annual journey around the sun, as it moves from equinox to solstice, solstice to equinox. We remind ourselves that Earth spins through a seasonal cycle of balance, activity, balance, and rest. Human beings were never designed to be perpetually calm or perpetually active. A healthy, fulfilling, and rewarding life will consist of action, activity, and stress; and this will be followed by downtime that allows us to de-stress and return to a neutral state, where healing can occur. To achieve anything in life and live according to our values, it is inevitable that we will have to endure periods of stress, uncertainty, and anxiety. This is *Karma Yoga*, the yoga of action.

In our yoga practice we can also use this template of balance, activity, balance, and rest. In our yoga asanas we achieve balance between effort (*sthira*) and relaxation (*sukha*). To stay strong and physically healthy, we must put a certain amount of stress upon our muscles and bones. However, too much stress and no relaxation and we risk damage from strain injuries. In a similar way, in our everyday lives we hope to achieve a healthy balance between relaxation and effort. To lead full and meaningful lives, we must be prepared to put up with a certain amount of stress as we take steps toward our goals. However, too much stress and no relaxation can result in burnout and stress-related illnesses, whereas too little stress and our lives risk becoming boring and unfulfilling.

One of the most precious gifts that yoga gives us is an ability to return to a neutral state. It is the state of balance between periods of activity. The practice of yoga enables us to drop down into a state where body and mind are at rest; this is a state of equanimity and equilibrium. It creates a space where the body and mind can realign and healing can occur. When you are in this place, the body and mind know what to do; the wisdom of body and mind flows freely like a river and the body can heal itself. Our yoga training shows us how we can get out of our own way and slip into this neutral state. Through our yoga practice, we can create the right conditions for this to happen, but it is not something that we can force: it is a state of grace.

Difficulties arise when we try to make permanent what is essentially a transitory state. Can any of us living in the world as it is maintain this yogic state of balance 24/7? Would we really want to? Yoga works best when it supports and enables us to live a rich, diverse, and fulfilling life. This will be a life filled with ups and downs, highs and lows, darkness and light, loss and gain, praise and blame, conflict and resolution of conflict. Yoga fails—or rather, we fail to use yoga skillfully—when we use it to escape or avoid life, when we try to create a bubble of serenity that exists in isolation from the wider world. Of course, naturally, sometimes we need time out from the fray of life, and our yoga and meditation practice can provide this. However, this is a temporary respite and then we must return to the fray. There is work to be done!

## Cultivating Your Yoga Garden

Like a garden, your yoga practice needs to be tended and cultivated if it is to grow and blossom. Spring is a good time to put some time and thought into planning what you would like to grow in your yoga garden so that it will give you pleasure all year round. Which seeds will you plant, and how will you feed, nourish, and water them so that they grow healthy and strong?

Sometimes over the winter your yoga practice can get a bit stagnant. If the problem is that you are still a bit sluggish after a long winter and not motivated to get onto your yoga mat, then try "rolling with resistance." Instead of arguing with yourself about why you *should* practice yoga, ask yourself, "What are the benefits to me of not practicing yoga?" Listen compassionately and non-judgmentally to the answers you come up with to this question, as they may well shed light on ways to get your yoga practice kick-started.

Here are some other questions that will help you to get your yoga garden growing again:

- What do I hope to get out of my yoga practice?
- What are the benefits of practicing yoga?
- What obstacles stand in the way of practicing yoga and how will I overcome them?

Above all be kind to yourself. If you spend a lot of time berating yourself for not practicing, you will begin to associate yoga with being nagged at! Be kind but firm. Remember how great yoga makes you feel; why would you deprive yourself of feeling that good? Look out for new green shoots.

Small is beautiful! When you spend five minutes a day weeding your garden, you can soon clear a space for planting spring flowers, and the same is true of your yoga practice. Look for small ways to integrate yoga into your daily life. For example, every time you check your phone, take a mindful breath in and out. Or spend a few minutes each day reading a yoga book or checking out yoga videos for ideas. Commit to five minutes of practice a day and watch your home yoga practice grow and blossom!

A journey of a thousand miles begins with a single step. However, a lack of confidence prevents many people from taking that first step and even starting yoga. Colin wants to take up yoga again. He's decided to wait until he's a bit fitter. He can no longer do many of the poses he used to be able to do, and he anticipates feeling embarrassed in class because he's not very flexible. He's also going to wait until he's lost a bit of weight.

He has been putting off re-joining his yoga class for a while now, waiting until he is good enough to join. Meanwhile, he is getting stiffer, his back aches, he gets breathless going upstairs, and he could really do with some yoga to sort him out!

The difficulty with the approach of waiting until you are perfect to join a class is that you could wait forever, as it is doing yoga that makes you more skilled and proficient at it. Like for any other activity, you must be prepared to do something "badly" before you can do it well. Mistakes are treasures and practice makes perfect. The Tao tells us, "A giant pine tree grows from a tiny sprout."[7] Today take a step toward your goal. Maybe the first step is just to go online and find out what classes are available in your area. And then the second step might be to email or phone the teacher. And before you know it, step by step, you've joined a class. To begin is the victory. The spring is the perfect time to take the plunge and try something new.

## Spring Equinox Yoga Practice

This spring equinox yoga practice has been designed to encapsulate the excitement and anticipation that comes with the arrival of spring. Poses such as the Runner's Lunge have been chosen to reflect a sense of being poised for action at the start of a race.

The magic of leaves unfurling, blossoms opening, and the world waking up after its winter sleep is reflected in the flowing sequence of Child's Pose into Upward-Facing Dog and back again. The exuberance of spring is expressed through poses such as Downward-Facing Dog with leg lifts.

We choose the balancing pose Warrior 3 to mirror day and night being perfectly balanced at the equinox. Stabilizing poses such as Chair Pose help us stay grounded as the energy of the year revs up.

The Standing Like a Tree Exercise and the Calming Cloud Meditation will help calm any restlessness and agitation brought on by the surge of growing season energy that comes with the changing season.

This practice is designed to be used around the time of the spring equinox, but it can be used all year round. It takes about 15 to 20 minutes. It is an energizing practice that also creates a sense of balance and stability. You will find at the end of these instructions an illustrated aide-mémoire for the whole practice.

---

7. Stephen Mitchell, trans., *Tao Te Ching: The Book of the Way* (London: Kyle Cathie, 2002), Tao 64.

## 1. Standing Like a Tree

Stand tall like a tree, feet parallel and about hip width apart, knees soft, face relaxed, shoulders down away from the ears. Your tailbone feels heavy, as though it is weighted, and the crown of your head is light and floats skyward. Imagine that there are roots going down from the soles of your feet deep into the earth. Picture in your mind's eye a tree in spring that you love or feel a connection to. (For more detailed instructions for this exercise, see page 22).

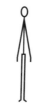

Standing Like a Tree

## 2. Warrior 1 Pose (*Virabhadrasana* 1)

Stand tall, feet hip width apart. Turn your right foot out slightly and take a big step forward with your left foot. Inhale while raising both arms above your head and bend the front knee over the ankle; exhale while lowering arms and straightening leg. Do 6 repetitions on this side, and on the final time stay for a few breaths with the arms raised. Then repeat on the other side.

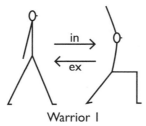

Warrior I

## 3a. Warrior 3 Pose (*Virabhadrasana* 3) variation

Before you go into either variation of this pose, silently repeat this affirmation: *I create balance in my life.*

Stand tall, feet hip width apart. Exhale as you tip your torso forward, at the same time raising one straight leg behind you, in line with your torso, and sweeping your arms out to the side like a bird's wings. Inhale and return to starting position. Repeat 4 times, holding the pose for a few breaths on the final time. Repeat on the other side.

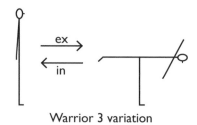

Warrior 3 variation

## 3b. Warrior 3 Pose (*Virabhadrasana* 3)

Stand tall, feet hip width apart and both arms above your head. Exhale as you tip your upper body forward, at the same time raising one straight leg behind you, in line with your torso, and keeping your raised arms in line with your ears (forming a human T-shape). Inhale and return to starting position. Repeat 4 times, holding the pose for a few breaths on the final time. Repeat on the other side.

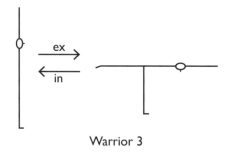

Warrior 3

## 4. Chair Pose (*Utkatasana*)

Stand tall, feet hip width apart and both arms above your head. Bend your knees and lower your bottom, as if to sit down on a high stool. Keep the ears between the arms and do not round the upper back. Imagine that your hips are being pulled downward and everything above the waist is reaching skyward. Stay for a few breaths. Inhale and imagine that you are drawing up energy from deep down in the earth into your power center at the belly. Exhale and imagine that this energy is pooling in the belly and recharging your battery. Come out of the pose by lowering your arms and straightening your legs.

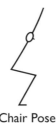

Chair Pose

## 5. Cat Pose (*Marjaryasana*) into Cow Pose (*Bitilasana*)

Start on all fours. Exhale and round the back up like an angry cat (*Marjaryasana*). Inhale into Cow Pose (*Bitilasana*), arching the back, lifting the chest up and away from the belly, and looking up slightly. Alternate between these two positions, rounding and arching the back. Repeat 6 times. (If you have a back problem, don't arch the back).

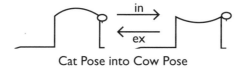

Cat Pose into Cow Pose

## 6. Runner's Lunge Pose (*Anjaneyasana*)

From Cat Pose (*Marjaryasana*), move one foot forward until it is between your hands. Come up onto your fingertips so that you can extend through the length of the spine. Do not round the upper back. Stay in the pose for a few breaths. As you stay in the pose, silently repeat this affirmation: *Inner wisdom guides my actions.* When you are ready, repeat the pose on the other side.

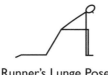

Runner's Lunge Pose

### 7. Downward-Facing Dog (*Adho Mukha Svanasana*) with leg lifts

From the Runner's Lunge Pose, turn the toes of the back foot under and step the front foot back into Downward-Facing Dog (*Adho Mukha Svanasana*). Establish yourself comfortably in Downward-Facing Dog, and then if you wish, lift one straight leg to hip height; if that feels okay, lift the leg higher so that it is in line with the torso. Do not tilt the pelvis. Repeat on the other side. Repeat 4 times on each side.

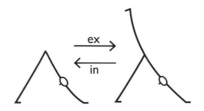

Downward-Facing Dog with Leg Lifts

### 8. Child's Pose (*Balasana*) into
### Upward-Facing Dog (*Urdhva Mukha Svanasana*)

From Downward-Facing Dog, bend the knees and sit back into Child's Pose (*Balasana*), arms outstretched along the floor. From Child's Pose, inhale and move forward into Upward-Facing Dog (*Urdhva Mukha Svanasana*), arching your back and keeping your knees on the floor. Exhale back into Child's Pose. Repeat 6 times. Each time you move into Upward-Facing Dog, silently repeat this affirmation: *I open to new possibilities.*

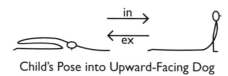

Child's Pose into Upward-Facing Dog

### 9. Child's Pose (*Balasana*) or Knees-to-Chest Pose (*Apanasana*)

Rest for a few breaths in either Child's Pose or Knees-to-Chest Pose (*Apanasana*).
    *If you are short of time, finish your practice here.*

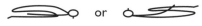
Child's Pose or Knees-to-Chest Pose

## 10. Calming Cloud Meditation

See instructions on page 36

Calming Cloud Meditation

## Spring Equinox Yoga Practice Overview

1. Standing Like a Tree.
2. Warrior 1 × 6 on each side. On final time stay for a few breaths with arms raised.
3a. Warrior 3 variation × 4 on each side. On final time stay for a few breaths. Affirmation: *I create balance in my life.*
3b. Warrior 3 × 4 on each side. On final time stay for a few breaths.
4. Chair Pose. Stay a few breaths.
5. Cat to Cow Pose × 6.
6. Runner's Lunge Pose. Stay for a few breaths. Affirmation: *Inner wisdom guides my actions.*
7. Downward-Facing Dog Pose with leg lifts × 4 on each side.
8. Child's Pose to Upward-Facing Dog × 6. Affirmation: *I open to new possibilities.*
9. Child's Pose or Knees-to-Chest Pose. Rest for a few breaths. *If you are short of time, finish your practice here.*
10. Calming Cloud Meditation.

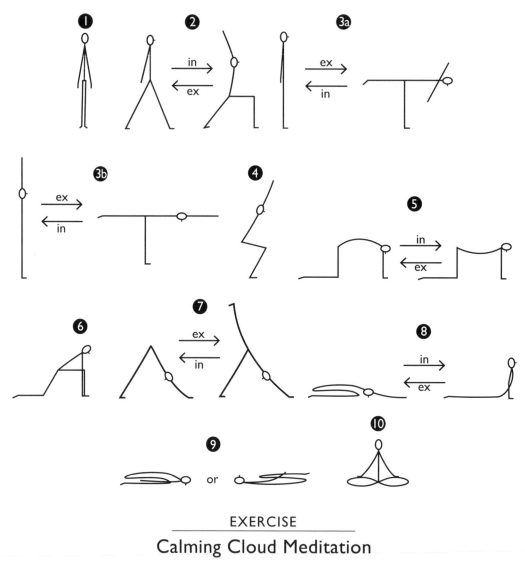

EXERCISE

## Calming Cloud Meditation

You can do this meditation at any time of year, but it is particularly good in spring when there is a surge of energy with the arrival of the growing season that can leave us feeling restless and agitated. This meditation is helpful for managing persistent, unwanted thoughts or at those times when you feel pressured or overwhelmed by anxiety. It calms an overactive mind, creating a sense of balance, freedom, and spaciousness.

Allow 10 minutes.

Find yourself a comfortable position, either sitting or lying. Notice where your body is in contact with the floor or your support, and allow your body to relax down into whatever is supporting you.

Let go of unnecessary tension; relax your shoulders down away from your ears and soften your face. If any part of your body feels tight or tense, then imagine that you are breathing into it on the inhale and letting go of any tension on the exhale.

Now imagine that you are somewhere where you can see the sky. A place where you feel safe, comfortable, and at ease. Notice the clear blue sky and notice any clouds that are passing through the sky. Remember that even when clouds cover the sky, there is still blue sky behind them.

Notice any thoughts or feelings that are coming into your mind. Imagine that each thought is like a cloud in the sky. If this thought were a cloud, what would it look like? Picture its shape, size, color, and texture. Notice that some clouds are white and fluffy, while others are dark and stormy.

Be aware of when you have been carried away by your thoughts. When this happens, congratulate yourself for noticing and once again start picturing your thoughts as clouds. We are not trying to get rid of thoughts, so you don't need to push clouds away. Simply let them drift across the sky in their own time.

Be aware of the temporary nature of clouds, how they come and go, and remember that behind the clouds there is always pure blue sky. Notice the space between one thought ending and another arising. The space between your thoughts is like the blue-sky space of pure consciousness. The spaciousness of the sky is the spaciousness of your mind, and the clouds are thoughts passing through the mind.

Now let go of picturing the sky and clouds. Bring your awareness back to your body lying or sitting here; notice where your body is in contact with the floor or your support. Become aware of your surroundings, noticing sounds inside the room and sounds outside of the room. Resolve to take this open, spacious, and accepting awareness into your everyday life and the next activity that you do today.

## Tree Wisdom in Spring

The perfect way to connect with the arrival of spring is to spend some time around trees, watching new life unfold. It's a joy to mindfully observe the signs of trees coming back to life with the appearance of catkins, leaves unfurling, and blossoms opening.

Seek out a tree and spend a few moments mindfully observing what signs of the arrival of spring you can see. Are the leaves coming into bud? Or have the leaves already reappeared on the tree? Can you see any birds or other wildlife on or around the tree? Are there any spring flowers growing around it? Use your senses to enjoy the moment: use your hands to touch the tree and enjoy the aroma of the tree, the colors, and the sounds that you can hear around you.

### EXERCISE
# Trees and Creativity during Spring

Once you have spent some mindful time around a tree, then use this as a springboard for your creativity. If you are stuck for ideas, here are some to get you going:

- Draw a bud coming into leaf, or draw any other part of the tree that interests you.
- Use colored pens, crayons, or paints to express how you feel about the tree.
- Set your timer for ten minutes and write meditatively about the tree, or write a poem or compose a song.
- If you are of an artistic bent and tend to shun science, then break this habit by finding out some info either about your tree or more generally the science behind the arrival of spring. Commit to fifteen minutes online reading up about this, read from a book in your local library, or talk to someone with a good knowledge of the subject. Once you have done this, observe whether your newfound knowledge adds to or detracts from your enjoyment of the season.
- If your chosen tree was a yoga pose, what shape would it take? Can you design a short yoga practice inspired by this tree?

**Meditation upon a Willow Tree at Spring Equinox**

Where I live, willow trees grow all along the banks of the river. In spring they are the first trees to come into leaf and yellow daffodils grow around them. The willow tree has taught me to listen to the wind whispering that spring is here. Below is the tree prose poem that I wrote in response to spending time meditatively around the willow.

*New leaves on the willow whisper to the wind that spring is here.*
*Moon in sky, sun on water, two white swans go sailing by. Old*
*bough bows down to the river, seeking willow mirrored there.*
*Wispy willow fronds reflected; river ripples willow hair. Blossom*
*on the wind is carried, wind whispers willow: spring is here.*

## Spring Equinox Meditation Questions

These questions are designed to be used around the time of the spring equinox. It's fine to use them a week or two before or after the actual date of the equinox. Guidance on how to use the seasonal meditation questions can be found in chapter 1.

- Over the coming season how will I go about growing healthy and loving relationships?
    - ᭡ Who is most important to me and how do I want to spend time with them this spring?
    - ᭡ What actions do I wish to take to support them and show them how much I care?
    - ᭡ How can I maintain a balance between giving and receiving love in my relationships?
    - ᭡ Are there any relationships in my life that need to be weeded out or pruned in order to create more time and energy for the people who really matter to me (including myself!)?
    - ᭡ Do I wish to plant seeds to grow new relationships?

- During the growing season, whatever we unite our energy with will expand and grow. How will I make best use of the fertile energy of the coming growing season?
    - ✧ Which projects do I wish to prioritize?
    - ✧ What lights my fire and what am I passionate about?
    - ✧ What actions will I need to take in order to ensure that the projects most dear to my heart come to fruition?
    - ✧ What should I say no to in order to create the space to say yes to the things that really matter to me? (What needs to be cut back or pruned?)
    - ✧ Who are my allies? Who can I enlist support from? Who shares my vision and will help me to make my dreams become a reality?

- How will I stay grounded during the busy growing season with its rampant, wild, fiery energy?
    - ✧ How will I stay in touch with my inner wisdom while taking outward action?
    - ✧ What will be my spiritual focus for this period?

- Night and day are perfectly balanced at the equinoxes. What steps do I need to take to restore balance to my life?
    - ✧ Are there any changes I need to make in my lifestyle to restore a good work-life balance?
    - ✧ How can I use my yoga practice as a way to bring balance into my life?

- How will I go about connecting with the natural world and appreciating the beauty of the season?
    - ✧ What signs of new growth and green shoots have I noticed in my surroundings and in my life?
    - ✧ Which seeds will I plant to bring, balance, hope, and beauty into my neighborhood and the various communities that I am a part of?
    - ✧ What actions, big or small, could I take to help and support the earth and its ecosystems?

# CHAPTER THREE

# Spring Turns to Summer

*End of April to mid-June in the Northern Hemisphere*
*End of October to mid-December in the Southern Hemisphere*

Spring to summer is a time of blossoming and unfolding. It is the height of the growing season, a fertile time, when whatever you unite your energy with will expand and grow. This is the perfect time to grow your yoga practice.

## Now Is the Time to Blossom

Between now and the summer solstice, the sun will reach the fullness of its waxing cycle, and then at the solstice the light will begin to wane again. So, we want to make the most of this short-lived fertile energy.

Our focus between now and the summer solstice is on outward achievements and action. Like a gardener, we decide which seeds to nurture so that they grow into strong and healthy plants. We decide which saplings to weed out to make space for our chosen plants to grow. Now is the time to bring your projects and ventures out into the light and watch them flourish.

This is a time to push rather than to yield. Do whatever it takes to make your heartfelt visions, dreams, and desires manifest in the world. Write emails, make phone calls, have conversations, and connect with those people who can help you to get your ideas out into the world. Ride the rising tide of growing season energy and make it happen. Be clear about what you want and go for it! At the same time the challenge of the season continues to be one of remembering to stay in touch with your inner wisdom while taking outward action. Your yoga practice can help you to stay grounded and not to get swept away by the fiery, rampant energy of the season.

In many cultures the arrival of summer, and its ensuing fertility, was celebrated through dance ritual. Dancing around the Maypole is a tradition that expresses the joyful exuberance of the season. The Maypole is said to symbolize the masculine aspect of God, the colorful ribbons are said to symbolize the feminine aspect, and the dance is their blissful union. This is a good time of year to incorporate elements of dance into your yoga practice.

In ancient times there were many myths that told of the Sun God and the Earth Goddess becoming lovers at this spring-summer time and their union ensuring nature's continuing fertility. It is a time for celebrating love, passion, sensuality, sexuality, and union of all kinds.

The spring and early summer are a time associated with youth. The beauty of yoga is that it allows you, whatever your actual age, to get in touch with that which is eternally youthful within. This is a good time to mentor a younger person as well as reconnect with the hopes, dreams, and aspirations of your younger self.

As spring changes to summer, nature is at her most creative; like a child with her first box of paints, she splashes bright colors everywhere. Every day some new miracle to feast our eyes upon. Nature unapologetically sings her song and always finds a way to blossom; even if you tarmac her over, she'll release a seed on the wind and hey presto, a wild flower appears through a crack in the pavement! We can imitate nature by getting in touch with our own creativity and using it to create magic in our life!

During the growing season, get sensual and use all your five senses to celebrate and enjoy the beauty of life. You could try the walking meditation included later in this chapter. Get out and about and enjoy your neighborhood. When out walking, be aware of the contact your feet make with the earth and remember to breathe. As you walk, feast your eyes on the riot of color as flowers open and blossom appears on the trees; smell the flowers; hear the bird song; taste the fruits of nature; touch and be touched by the world around you. Sensuality is the art of everyday ecstasy!

## Sensuality, Sexuality, and Ecstasy (*Samadhi*)

Sexuality and sensuality are at the forefront of our awareness during the spring to summer period, when nature is entering her most fertile period. Traditionally, the rites of spring and summer celebrate the union of lovers. The heavenly union of sun and earth was often imitated in spring-summer rituals, and courting couples collected blossoms in the woods and lit fires in the evening. Lovers would leap over the fire, and there were nights of lovemaking in the fields to ensure the fertility and fruitfulness of the land.

During spring to summer, nature's creations, such as blossoms, have a luminescent quality that can inspire our yoga practice, bringing us closer to the yogic state of clarity and light (*sattva*). This sattvic state mirrors the state of enlightenment (*samadhi*), when the "object" of meditation and the meditator become one. However, to stay grounded we will also need to harness a heavier (*tamas*) energy to prevent us from being swept away by the frenetic (*rajas*) energy of the season. It is important to remember that *samadhi* is not a practice; it is a state of grace.

Part one of Patanjali's Yoga Sutras is entitled "Chapter on Ecstasy." Patanjali taught that the ecstatic state (*samadhi*) is the fruit of a disciplined yoga practice and is achieved by completely severing ties with world of material nature (*prakriti*) and dwelling in the spirit self (*purusha*). The liberated being then exists in a state of eternal freedom and aloneness (*kaivalya*). Whereas Patanjali envisaged spiritual liberation as a disembodied, isolated state, in Seasonal Yoga we conceive of ecstasy as being available in the here and now on earth. Through our connection to the beauty of the changing seasons, we become as one with the world: we are part of it all.

In the dualistic outlook of *Classical Yoga*, the world of matter is considered impure and that of spirit pure. The circle of sexuality is both beautiful and messy, with a definite biological element to it. Women were labeled closer to nature, and their experience of menstruation, pregnancy, and birth were deemed impure states.[8] Once again, this is an example of how as modern-day yoga practitioners we must reinvent yoga, especially in support of women.

When we consider that the aim of Classical Yoga was to reach a state of enlightenment by detaching from the material world, we can understand, from this point of view, why celibacy (*brahmacarya*) was advocated. Whether a relationship is going well and

---

8. Lynn Teskey Denton, *Female Ascetics in Hinduism* (Albany: State University of New York Press, 2004), 25.

you are madly in love, or it is going badly and you are heartbroken, intimate relations inevitably disturb one's yogic calm!

However, celibacy isn't an easy one to sell, and most yoga teachers nowadays interpret *brahmacarya* as acting in a sexually responsible way. It is certainly an issue worth debating, especially with the advent of online dating apps, where your next partner is only a scroll away and can be chosen like a dish on the menu. It is also essential that yoga organizations ensure that rigorous procedures are in place to protect the vulnerable from sexual harassment or abuse, and that individual practitioners, particularly those in positions of authority and power, act in a sexually respectful and responsible way.

Our sexual relationships can provide us with the greatest highs and lows of our life. The old cliché that it is better to have loved and lost than never to have loved at all still stands for most of us. So if we decide to immerse ourselves in the messy, beautiful roller-coaster ride of relationships, our challenge is how our yoga practice and a yogic way of life can help us skillfully ride the ups and downs of intimacy.

Sometimes love can be easy and spontaneous, and at other times, like most good things in life, it has to be worked at. So many different aspects of our life, including the more mundane (but vital) aspects such as contraception, are encircled by sexuality. By developing our awareness of the changing seasons and our yoga practice, we can become familiar with the wisdom of our own rhythms and cycles (including the menstrual cycle). In this way we can heal the schism between spirituality and sexuality, and once again heaven and earth are reunited.

Our physical yoga practice can certainly give us a flexibility and stamina that can enhance our sexual relationships. And our mindfulness practice enables us to give our partner, and ourselves, the gift of being fully present to the experience of lovemaking. And an awareness of the breath allows us to relax into the experience and open to our bliss.

Over a lifetime, at various times, we may or may not be in a sexual relationship. However, sensual enjoyment is always available to us. Whether we are happily or unhappily in a relationship will often depend on circumstances beyond our control; in contrast, whatever our circumstances, we can always choose to mindfully use our five senses to appreciate the beauty of the season and fall head over heels in love with life again.

## Celebrating the Dance of Life

Spring to summer is a sensual time when new life is unfolding all around us. Sunlight kisses the earth and the earth responds by blossoming. I love to observe how people unfold and blossom as their yoga practice progresses. Some people, when they first come to yoga, are tight and prickly, like a hedgehog curled up in a ball. It is a privilege to see them blossom as their yoga practice teaches them how to dance with life again.

In Hindu tradition the world is danced into being by gods and goddesses. As spring changes to summer, nature is dancing a sensual dance of creation, and the world is coming into bloom. Now is the time to dance your light into being, manifesting it in the world. We are all part of the dance of life. On a macrocosmic scale there is the dance of the sun, moon, and earth, which gives us night and day, the tides, and the seasons. On a smaller scale there is the dance of our daily lives lived out through the seasons of our lives.

Dance can be a way of honoring both sensuality and sexuality. In many cultures dance marked the various transition points of life. There were courtship dances, fertility dances, and dances to prepare for giving birth. Dance can be a meditation and lead to ecstatic states in which the dancer and the dance become one. The dancer is no longer dancing; rather, she is being danced. I like to imagine that had yoga been handed down to us over the millennia from mother to daughter as well as from father to son, it would include some element of sacred dance.

Dance is sensual and can be a great way of getting your creative juices flowing. Yoga and dance combine to make great partners. Try using dance as a warm-up for your yoga practice. Put on your favorite dance music and just allow yourself to be danced. Make this into a dancing meditation by focusing your awareness on the sound of the music, the sensations of your body moving, and the dance of your own breath. Feel those happy hormones soar! Flowing yoga sequences (*vinyasa*) also have a very dance-like quality. The Salute to the Sun (*Surya Namaskar*) is a fiery sun dance, combining wave-like movements with breath awareness. The Dancer Pose (*Natarajasana*) is of course the perfect asana to include in your dance-inspired *vinyasa*.

## Spring to Summer Yoga Practice

As spring changes to summer, the whole world is coming into bloom, and it is the theme of blossoming that has inspired this practice. That sense of opening and flowering is conveyed through expansive poses such as Warrior 1 and Bow Pose.

This is a time associated with dancing, and so naturally the Dancer Pose is included. It's also a time traditionally connected with the flowering of sexuality, and the Pelvic Flower exercise has been chosen to reflect this.

This practice is designed to be used during the spring to early summer period; however, it's fine to use it any time of year. It will help you cultivate an open, expansive attitude. It will enhance your ability to embrace and dance with life. And encourage you to blossom to your full potential.

Allow 20 to 30 minutes.

### 1. Standing Like a Tree in Blossom

Stand tall like a tree. (Or, if you prefer, this exercise can be done sitting in a straight-backed chair). Your feet are parallel and about hip width apart, knees soft, face relaxed, shoulders down away from the ears; your tailbone feels heavy as though it is weighted, and the crown of your head feels light and floats skyward.

Now picture the beauty of a tree in blossom. Notice its shape, the blossom's color, its fragrance. Stay here for a few breaths, enjoying the beauty of the image of the tree.

*For a longer version: see the Visualizing a Tree in Blossom exercise that follows this yoga practice.*

Standing Like a Tree in Blossom

## 2. Knee to chest into Dancer Pose (*Natarajasana*) variation

Stand tall, feet hip width apart, arms by your sides. Hug the right knee into your chest, and then take the right leg behind you and catch hold of the ankle with the right hand. Lower the foot back to the floor and repeat on the other side. Repeat 10 times on each side.

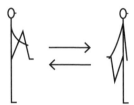

Knee to chest into Dancer Pose variation

## 3. Dancer Pose (*Natarajasana*) variation

Stand tall, feet hip width apart, arms by your sides. Bend your right knee and with your right hand catch hold of your ankle. Take the left arm either out to the side at shoulder height or above the head. Stay for a few breaths and then repeat on the left side.

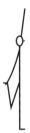

Dancer Pose variation

## 4. Warrior 1 (*Virabhadrasana* 1) variation

Stand tall, feet hip width apart, arms by your sides. Turn your left foot slightly out and take a big step forward with your right leg. Inhale and bend your front, right knee, opening your arms out wide to the side, picturing a blossom opening. Exhale, straighten your right leg, and lower your arms back to your sides, picturing the blossom closing back to bud. Do 6 repetitions on this side and then repeat on the other side.

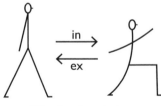

Warrior I variation

## 5. Dancer Pose (*Natarajasana*)

Come into Dancer Pose variation (from step 3), and from here tip the torso forward, extending the back foot away from you and reaching forward and up with the opposite arm. Stay for a few breaths and then repeat on the other side. If you have balance problems, practice facing a wall with your extended hand resting on the wall for support.

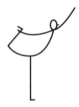

Dancer Pose

## 6. Puppy Dog Pose (*Uttana Shishosana*) and Child's Pose (*Balasana*)

Come onto all fours. Walk the hands forward along the floor until your arms, head, and torso form one, long diagonal line, keeping the thighs at a 90-degree angle. Keep the ears between the arms. Stay here for a few breaths. Then bend the knees and sit the bottom back onto the heels and rest for a few breaths in Child's Pose (*Balasana*).

*For a shorter practice, end here.*

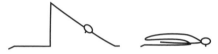

Puppy Dog Pose and Child's Pose

## 7. Bow Pose (*Dhanurasana*) variation

Lie face down on the floor, arms by your sides. Inhale and lift your chest, bending both knees. Exhale, lower your chest, and straighten your legs back to the floor. Repeat 6 times and stay in the final pose for a few breaths.

*If you wish to work at a gentler level, then skip the next pose, Bow Pose* (Dhanurasana), *and go straight to Child's Pose* (Balasana) *in step 9 or repeat the Bow Pose variation of step 7 once more.*

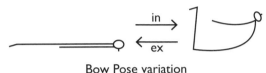

Bow Pose variation

## 8. Bow Pose (*Dhanurasana*)

Lie on your front, arms by your sides. Bend both knees and catch hold of your ankles. Lift your chest and knees up and away from the floor; gently pulling your shoulders back to open the chest. If comfortable, stay here for a few breaths. Then lower down to the floor, release the ankles, straighten your legs along the floor, and turn your head to one side, resting for a few breaths.

Bow Pose

## 9. Child's Pose (*Balasana*)

Rest here for a few breaths.

Child's Pose

## 10. Pelvic Flower Exercise

It's important to keep the pelvic floor strong, but at the same time it's also important to know how to relax it. This exercise will help you relax the pelvic floor and can also enhance sexual enjoyment.

Lie on your back in Supine Butterfly Pose (*Supta Baddha Konasana*). Rest your hands either on your belly or above your head. For comfort, prop your knees on bolsters, cushions, or blocks. Imagine there is a beautiful flower between your legs, at the pelvic floor. As you inhale the flower opens, and as you exhale the flower closes back to bud. Repeat for a few breaths. Be present to any sensations that arise in the pelvic floor area as you do this exercise. Then bring the knees together in to Knees-to-Chest Pose (*Apanasana*) and relax here for a few breaths.

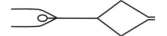

Pelvic Flower Exercise

## 11. Full-Body Stretch
Take your arms overhead and stretch your legs out. Lengthen tall along the floor.

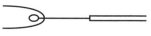

Full-Body Stretch

## 12. Visualizing a Tree in Blossom
See instructions on page 52.

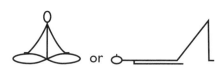

Visualizing a Tree in Blossom

## Spring to Summer Yoga Practice Overview
1. Standing Like a Tree in Blossom.
2. Knee to chest into Dancer Pose variation × 10 on each side.
3. Dancer Pose variation. Stay for a few breaths. Repeat on other side.
4. Warrior 1 variation × 6. Inhale: picture blossom opening. Exhale: picture blossom closing back to bud. Repeat on other side.
5. Dancer Pose. Stay for a few breaths. Repeat on other side.

6. Puppy Dog Pose. Stay for a few breaths. Rest in Child's Pose. *For a shorter practice, end here.*

7. Bow Pose variation × 6. Stay in final pose for a few breaths. *For a gentler practice, skip step 8 or repeat this step in its place.*

8. Bow Pose. Stay for a few breaths.

9. Child's Pose. Rest here for a few breaths.

10. Pelvic Flower Exercise in Supine Butterfly Pose. Inhale: picture a flower opening at the pelvic floor. Exhale: picture the flower closing back to bud.

11. Full-Body Stretch. Lengthen tall along floor.

12. Visualizing a Tree in Blossom.

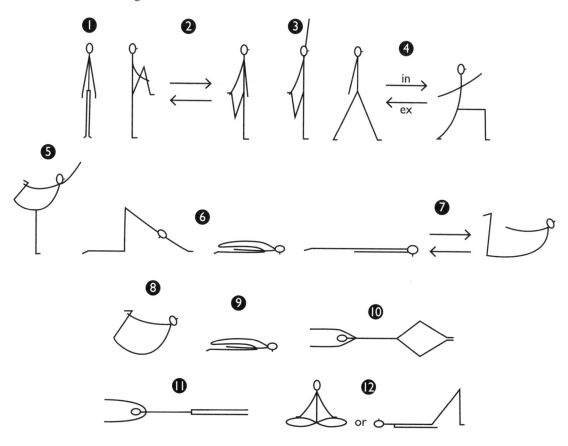

# Visualizing a Tree in Blossom

Focusing on the natural beauty of a tree in blossom has an uplifting effect and will help you to feel a peaceful sense of connection to the natural world. This exercise can be done sitting or lying down.

Picture the beauty of a tree in blossom. Notice its shape, colors, and fragrance. Now imagine that you *are* a tree in blossom. Feel the space around you, the blue sky above you, and the earth below you. Picture your roots going deep down into the soil, spreading, wrapping around rocks and boulders, giving you strength, nourishment, and stability. Feel yourself receiving energy from the warm sun. Allow yourself to be breathed. You are a tree in blossom breathing. You are part of it all. You are a tree, connected to the earth, the sky, the air, and the sunshine. Stay here for a few more breaths, feeling your connection to the intricate web of life.

When you are ready, let go of the image of the tree in blossom. Become aware of where your body is in contact with the floor or your support. Become aware of your surroundings. Take this peaceful feeling of connectedness into the next thing that you do today.

# The Loving Kindness Walking Meditation

Spring-to-summer time is often associated with romantic love. The following meditation helps cultivate a more universal sense of loving kindness for both ourselves and others.

Walking meditation can be done any time of year but is particularly good in spring and summer, especially at those times when you feel torn between the urge to do some yoga and the desire to get out in the sunshine. It's ideal when you want to meditate but don't want to spend more time sitting. It gets you out of your head and into your body, calming and clearing the mind, relieving and releasing stress. It grounds you, strengthening your connection to your surroundings and the earth. It boosts circulation and lifts your mood.

Whether you are walking in an urban or rural setting, try to find beauty and tranquility wherever you are. At the same time stay safe, aware of your surroundings, and alert to any hazards, such as traffic and so on.

Allow 10 to 20 minutes for this meditation

Start the meditation by walking and simply paying attention to the physical sensations associated with walking. Particularly be aware of the sensations in your feet and "walk as if your feet are kissing the earth."[9]

Next begin to send yourself love and good wishes as you walk. Wish yourself well by silently repeating phrases such as *I hope you have a good day. I hope things go well for you today.* Or if you prefer, you can use formal loving kindness (*metta*) phrases as you walk:

> *May I be safe.*
> *May I be happy.*
> *May I be healthy.*
> *May I live with ease.*[10]

Or you can shorten the phrases to *safe, happy, healthy,* and *ease.* Use one word with each step that you take.

If any self-criticism arises, surround that with love too. Have compassion for any difficulties that you are experiencing today, or if you are feeling happy, then allow yourself to fully enjoy those happy feelings too.

Next start sending out good wishes to passersby. Try to see the good within each person that you pass. Notice any critical judgments that you make about people. Recognize your shared humanity and acknowledge that for them, like for you, life isn't always easy. Silently repeat phrases for them such as *I hope you have a good day. I hope things go well for you today.*

Or, if you prefer, you can use formal loving kindness (*metta*) phrases as you walk. You can strengthen your sense of connection with them by silently repeating phrases for both of you: *May you and I be happy. May you and I live with ease.*

---

9. Thich Nhat Hanh, *The Long Road Turns to Joy: A Guide to Walking Meditation* (Berkeley, CA: Parallax Press, 2011), 67.

10. Christopher K. Germer, *The Mindful Path to Self-Compassion: Freeing Yourself from Destructive Thoughts and Emotions* (New York: The Guilford Press, 2009), 184–186.

You can also widen your circle of compassion by sending good wishes to animals, trees, the river, the air, birds, and the earth.

To conclude your walking meditation, bring your awareness back to observing the sensations of your feet in contact with the earth as you walk. Thank the earth for supporting you during this walking meditation.

## Tree Wisdom: Spring to Summer

Spring to summer is a time of blossoming. Trees offer us the perfect way of connecting to the beauty that is blossoming during this season.

When you are out and about, be on the lookout for trees in blossom and take a few moments to mindfully enjoy the tree's beauty. Use your senses to appreciate this precious moment; enjoy the colors, textures, smells, and sounds of the scene. Look closely at an individual blossom flower and observe the intricacy of its construction.

Close your eyes and picture the tree in blossom, and then open your eyes and look at the tree again. Recall the image later in your day to induce a sense of calm contemplation.

### EXERCISE

## Trees and Creativity during Spring to Summer

After having mindfully spent time enjoying a tree in blossom, you can use this as a springboard for your creativity. If you are stuck for ideas, here are some to get you going:

- Mindfully take some photos of a tree in blossom. Use them as screen savers and enjoy a peaceful moment each time you look at them. Or if you have access to a printer, print out some photos and place them in locations that will remind you to stop and enjoy their beauty.
- Do an online search and find paintings, poems, prose, songs, or photos around the theme of *blossom*. Spend a few moments mindfully enjoying your discoveries.
- How much do you know about the science of blossoming? What is it that makes a tree put so much energy into producing this spectacular display?

Commit to fifteen minutes of online reading up about this, read from a book in your local library, or talk to someone with a good knowledge of the subject. Once you have done this, observe whether your newfound knowledge adds or detracts from your enjoyment of the season.

- Take a small amount of blossom from a tree, without damaging the tree, and use it as a focus for meditation either informally, just stopping to look at it mindfully when you pass by, or for a more formal sitting meditation: have the blossom where you can fix your gaze upon it and when your mind wanders, gently bring it back to observing the blossom. Then sit for a few quiet moments holding the image of the blossom in your mind's eye.
- Try out the spring to summer yoga practice in this chapter, which has a theme of blossoming and includes a Tree in Blossom visualization.

## Meditation upon an Apple Tree in Blossom

One day last spring I was walking through parkland, bordered by some wasteland that used to be the town rubbish tip, and a young apple tree bathed in sunshine caught my eye. I'd never noticed this little tree before, but it looked so beautiful in full blossom, glowing golden in the sunshine. It seemed poignant to me that such beauty could grow out of the ugliness of what had been a rubbish dump. This tree taught me about staying effortlessly in touch with that which is light, pure, beautiful, and graceful within and how it is possible to blossom even in a world that is neither perfect nor pure. Below is the tree prose poem that I wrote in response to meditatively spending time around the apple tree.

> *Apple tree in blossom, you are the Tree of Life; your roots go down through oceans of fire to the Center of the World; your branches grow up through sky and space to hold up the heavens. Full moon smiles down through your branches; new moon brings you baby buds. Sunlight; and star-shaped flowers open; five white petals tinged with pink. Weave a crown of love from blossomed branches; your generosity knows no bounds. Happiness is your sweet-scented petals, confetti carried on the breeze. Tree in blossom, you are breathing; tree in blossom being breathed.*

# Spring to Summer Meditation Questions

These questions are designed to be used any time from around the end of April to mid-May in the Northern Hemisphere and from around the end of October to mid-November in the Southern Hemisphere. Guidance on how to use the seasonal meditation questions can be found in chapter 1.

- The spring to summer period is a time of blossoming. What do I wish to grow and blossom in my life at this time?
  - ↬ Who helps me blossom and fulfill my potential?
  - ↬ Which relationships do I want to celebrate?
  - ↬ Who do I feel passionate about? Who lights my fire? Who inspires me?

- Between now and the summer solstice is a very fertile time. How will I best use this short-lived fertile period?
  - ↬ What do I want to achieve?
  - ↬ Which projects do I want to grow and blossom?
  - ↬ What are my priorities and what is most important to me?
  - ↬ What heartfelt actions do I need to take in order to ensure these projects come to fruition?
  - ↬ What needs pruning or cutting back in order to create the space for healthy growth?
  - ↬ Who shares my vision and how can I enlist their support to make my dreams become a reality?

- At this fiery, fertile, active time how will I use my yoga practice to stay grounded?

- Are there disconnected parts of my life that need to be reunited in order that I might become healthy and whole again?

- Spring to summer is a time associated with youth and the young.
  - ↬ Is there a younger person in my life whom I can help and support?

↬ When with younger people, do I maintain a good balance between talking and imparting wisdom to them and listening to and learning from them?

- During spring and summer, nature is at her most creative.
    - ↬ Have I any hidden talents that have not yet been developed or realized?
    - ↬ Is there a particular gift or talent that I would like to cultivate or nurture?
    - ↬ What small steps could I take to develop this talent?

- At this fertile time when all around is blossoming, how do I honor my own sexuality?
    - ↬ How do I celebrate my body and reject body-shaming messages from the media?
    - ↬ How do I help and support others to do the same?

- The earth is so generous and bountiful at this time. How can I give back to the earth?
    - ↬ Are there any small steps I could take this season to improve my neighborhood or to make it more beautiful?
    - ↬ Can I inspire others to take small steps to protect the environment?

- How will I enjoy the beauty of the season using all my senses? How can I fall in love with life again?

CHAPTER FOUR

# Summer Solstice

*June 20–23 in the Northern Hemisphere*
*December 20–23 in the Southern Hemisphere*

The summer solstice is a doorway into the second half of the year. It is a fiery, fertile, exuberant, passionate time, when the earth's loveliness just seems to go on and on. Energy-wise the summer solstice is like the full moon; it is pregnant with possibility.

## The Sun Bows Down to the Moon at the Summer Solstice

At the summer solstice the sun has ripened to its fullness and the earth is at her most fertile and productive. It is a peak time that can be compared to ovulation within the menstrual cycle. Now the earth is as ripe as the full moon, and she dazzles us with her ability to give birth to beauty: blossoms in the sunshine, the perfume of honeysuckle blown on the breeze, swallows swooping and diving through a clear blue sky, and fruit ripening on the bush. In some traditions motherhood and the mother aspect of the Goddess are honored at this fertile time.

It is a dual celebration: as well as celebrating the power of the sun, we are also welcoming back the darkness. The expansion of the light, which began at the winter solstice in December, reaches its fullness at the summer solstice, and thereafter the sun's powers will begin to wane. The year has turned and gradually the days will begin to get shorter and the nights longer. The waxing cycle of the darkness has begun.

At the summer solstice there is a shift in the earth's energy. We are moving from sun to moon, yang to yin, light to dark, sunlight to shadow, fire to water, action to contemplation, and outer to inner. Once we have accepted and relaxed into this transition, it is rich with possibilities. Between now and the winter solstice is the time to incubate ideas, spending time considering which seeds we wish to nurture in the dark half of the year, ready to send up new green shoots next spring. The second half of the year is not a time for action; it is a time for dreaming our ideas into being, and our yoga practice can support and enhance this self-reflection.

It is natural to want summer to go on forever, and many of us feel pangs of regret that it won't. And although summer isn't over yet, there are still warm, sunny days ahead; yet at the same time the year has turned, and gradually the days will shorten and the nights get longer. At the winter solstice in December we wholeheartedly celebrate the return of the sun and the rebirth of the light; however, at the summer solstice, we may feel more ambivalent about welcoming back the waxing cycle of the darkness. We balance this by remembering that the dark half of the year gives us the opportunity to take stock, to plan, and to gestate ideas, ready to be delivered out into the world during next spring and summer's growing season.

At the solstice the sun appears to stand still before it changes direction. We too stand still, pause, and take time to reflect. We have reached the top of a mountain and stop now to take in the view. We look back over the journey we have taken since the winter solstice and look ahead to the path that leads us into the darker half of the year.

## Thank You, Sunlight; Thank You, Shadow

Although we enthusiastically welcome back the sun at the winter solstice, it somehow goes against the grain to celebrate the return of the darkness at the summer solstice. The sun is a star at the center of our solar system; its light powers the photosynthesis that plants need to grow, and plants in turn give us the food and oxygen that we need to breathe. The sun has a lot going for it, and it's easy to see why we should celebrate its powers at the solstices, whereas advocating celebrating the return of the darkness at the summer solstice is a harder sell!

Fear of darkness seems to be built into our DNA. This makes sense when you consider that before the advent of electricity, when night fell, there would have been total darkness. The darkness of night naturally would have struck a chord of fear into our ancestors, as in darkness they were vulnerable to attack. Those starry nights when the full moon lit up the night sky must have been precious and welcome.

Culturally, religiously, and in our psyche, the light has come to be associated with goodness, and darkness with evil. However, when we demonize darkness, we miss out on the healing, nurturing qualities that darkness brings. So many good things happen in the dark: a baby grows in the darkness of the womb, a seed begins life in the darkness of the soil, the darkness embraces us and gives us rest at the end of each day. The darkness offers a refuge where we can rest, sleep, and dream. Sunlight and shadow create balance in our lives. Light without shade becomes harsh, relentless, and overpowering. In our towns and cities light pollution confuses birds and animals and disturbs our own circadian rhythms.

During the first half of the year, between the winter and summer solstice, when the light is expanding, our focus is upon action, achievement, and getting things done. At this time we follow a path that spirals from our center outward into the world. Now, at the summer solstice, as the light begins to wane, we change direction and turn to face the path that spirals back into our center. We welcome back the dark half of the year because it gives us the opportunity to rest, recuperate, and regenerate after the frenetic activity of the growing season. We begin a return journey home to a peaceful place within, where we can find solace and regeneration. Now is the time to bring our outward achievements inside, to a place of sanctuary, so they can be processed and transformed.

The yogic concept of withdrawal becomes relevant at the summer solstice when we gradually turn from an active, outward focus to an inner, more contemplative focus. Withdrawal of the senses (*pratyahara*) is the fifth of Patanjali's eight limbs of yoga (Yoga Sutras 2.54, 2.55).[11] It involves training the senses to quieten down and not to get carried away by outside stimuli. Other yoga texts compare yogic withdrawal to a tortoise withdrawing its limbs into its shell. Withdrawal prepares the yogi for the last three limbs of yoga: concentration, meditation, and pure contemplation.

11. Barbara Stoler Miller, *Yoga: Discipline of Freedom; The Yoga Sutra Attributed to Patanjali* (New York: Bantam Books, 1998), 59.

There is to be found, within each of us, an island that is our refuge from the storm. We all know this place, and we all know how to find it, although we may have temporarily forgotten how. It is our birthright. Maybe your way of accessing this place is through yoga and meditation, or perhaps you find it when you're gardening, dancing, running, listening to music, making scones, making love, or daydreaming. It's good to practice coming home to this place when times are calm, because then when stormy weather arrives, it will be available to you.

At the summer solstice, as the year turns, we are given a chance to pause and reflect, both on our outer journey since the winter solstice and on how we wish to use the inner journey that lies ahead in the darker half of the year. By working with the ebb and flow of the year in this way, we balance shadow and sunlight in our lives—our inner and outer lives, private and public, and activity and rest. In this way we create the conditions for a healthy and wholesome way of life.

## The Earth as Mother at the Summer Solstice

Mother Earth is parent to us all. We come from earth and eventually return to earth. She is the ground we walk upon—supporting us, providing us with food and shelter, giving us water when we are thirsty and rest when we are tired. She is a gentle, kind, loving mother and at the same time she is also a fierce mother who can kill us with earthquakes, tornadoes, hurricanes, and erupting volcanoes. She is to be loved, respected, and feared!

The Indian Goddess *Kali Ma* mirrors this dual aspect of earth as both creator and destroyer. She is the Hindu Triple Goddess of creation, preservation, and destruction and is known as the Dark Mother. In the West she is mainly known as a destructive goddess. However, in India she is also recognized primarily as the fount of all love and compassion (*karuna*), and this compassion flows into the world through women, who are her agents on earth.[12] The goddess Kali Ma is a wonderful metaphor for the passage of the seasons that also go through a cycle of creation, preservation, destruction, and rebirth. At the summer solstice the very moment when we celebrate the sun's fullness is also the pivotal point when the sun's powers start to wane.

Kali Ma also sometimes manifests as *Durga*, a warrior queen who personifies the fighting spirit of a mother protecting her young. As the goddess of both creation and destruc-

---

12. Barbara G. Walker, *The Women's Encyclopedia of Myths and Secrets* (New York: Harper Collins, 1983), 490.

tion, Kali Ma provides a good metaphor for the complexity of feelings that we have, both as a society and as individuals, toward our mothers and the concept of motherhood.

Our religious and spiritual organizations, including yoga, have a deficit of experience if they have been created exclusively by those who have no experience of menstruation, pregnancy, giving birth, breastfeeding, or even childcare responsibilities. Our challenge now is, how do we reclaim and reintegrate this essential feminine part of human experience and bring it back into the mainstream of our spiritual life?

The summer solstice is a good time to explore how you feel about your own experience of being mothered, how you feel about parenting (or choosing not to be a parent), and how to go about "mothering" yourself. How you reflect on fertility and motherhood will depend on which season of your life you are in. For some of us creativity is expressed through physically giving birth and parenting children, while others make a positive, conscious decision not to have children at all, preferring to nurture, sustain, and protect life in other ways.

Learning how to "mother" ourselves well is an essential part of our spiritual practice. Of course, we must also remember that nurturing, nourishing, and caring skills are not exclusive to one gender. If we are to be good enough parents, to our children and our grown-up children, then it is essential that we learn to model good self-care to them.

Below are some ideas on how to incorporate this component of nurturing and nourishing into your yoga practice:

- At the start of your yoga session, imagine that you are drawing a circle of light around yourself. This is a circle of safety and protection. Consciously place your everyday concerns and preoccupations on the outside of the circle.

- During your practice, monitor your internal dialogue. Is it harsh and self-critical? If so, cultivate a way of talking to yourself that is kind and compassionate. In this way you will always feel welcomed when you step onto your yoga mat.

- Like a loving mother, give yourself the gift of presence. Be present to and aware of bodily sensations, thoughts passing through the mind, and feelings as they arise; respond accordingly by adjusting your practice with kindness.

- Above all be aware of the breath, as the breath is the umbilical cord that connects us to life itself.

Like a loving parent, we can create a safe and supportive yoga environment within which we feel safe and confident enough to take risks, make mistakes, and so develop and grow. When we feel supported and cared for in this way, we will want to return to our practice often, as it is sweet like mother's milk.

## Three Mother Mantras to Nurture and Nourish You

*Ma, Om,* and *Sa'ham* are three nurturing and nourishing mantras that can be incorporated into your yoga practice. Mantras are an excellent way of stilling the mind and uplifting the spirit. They can be vocalized or silently repeated.

### The Mantra *Ma*

Repetition of the mantra *Ma* induces a sense of well-being and connectedness. *Ma* is the basic mother syllable of Indo-European languages. In the Far East *Ma* represents the "spark of life" and was often defined as intelligence.[13]

### The Mantra *Om*

In the Upanishads the mantra *Om* is referred to as "the supreme syllable, the mother of all sound," and sound was the Great Goddess's tool of creation. The meaning of *Om* was something like "pregnant belly." *Om* was the *mantra matrika,* the Mother of Mantras, and is considered to be the first of all the creative spells spoken by the Goddess to bring the world into being.[14]

### The Mantra *Sa'ham*

*Sa'ham* can be translated as "she I am." It was conceived by Tantric poets who worshipped Kali Ma as the Mother and the basis of all creation: "All is the Mother and She is reality herself."[15] This yogic mantra is pronounced *so-hum* and is said to be the sound

---

13. Barbara G. Walker, *The Woman's Encyclopedia of Myths and Secrets* (New York: Harper Collins 1983), 560.

14. Barbara G. Walker, *The Woman's Dictionary of Symbols and Sacred Objects* (New York: Harper Collins, 1988), 99.

15. Barbara G. Walker, *The Woman's Encyclopedia of Myths and Secrets* (New York: Harper Collins, 1983), 490.

made naturally with each inhalation and exhalation. The in-breath naturally makes a *so* sound, and the exhale naturally makes a *hum* sound. *Sa'ham* can also be translated as "I am that."

## Summer Solstice Yoga Practice

This practice enables you to stand still, pause, and regather your energy following the busy activity of the growing season. We use *asanas* such as Tortoise Pose (*Kurmasana*) to honor the change of direction initiated at the summer solstice from outward activity to inner contemplation.

The summer solstice is a time associated with earth as mother, and we use the mantras *Ma* and *Om* to nurture and nourish.

The practice is inspired by and designed to be used around the time of the summer solstice. It's also fine to use it any time of year. It has a calming effect and is perfect for those hyper-busy times when you need to withdraw from the world to regather yourself. It is the go-to cooling practice for hot summer days when you don't want to do anything too energetic.

Allow 15 to 20 minutes.

### 1. Mantra *Ma* and Arm Movements

Find a comfortable seated position. Rest your hands on your belly. Inhale and take your arms out to the side. Exhale and bring your hands back to the belly, chanting the mantra *Ma*. Stay for one breath, with the hands resting on the belly. Repeat 6 times.

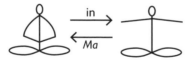

Mantra *Ma* and Arm Movements

### 2. *Ma-Om* Kneeling Sequence

Come to tall kneeling, hands in the Prayer Position (*Namaste*). Inhale and raise your arms. Exhale and fold forward into Child's Pose (*Balasana*), with arms outstretched along the floor. Inhale and come onto all fours. On the exhale, chanting *Om*, sit back into Child's Pose. Inhale and come back to tall kneeling with arms raised. Exhale and bring your hands into prayer position. Repeat the sequence 4 to 6 times.

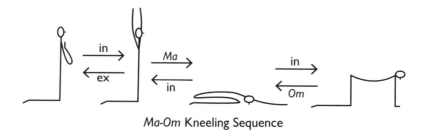

Ma-Om Kneeling Sequence

### 3. Seated Forward Bend (*Paschimottanasana*)

Sit tall, legs outstretched (bend the knees to ease the pose). Inhale and raise your arms. Exhale and fold forward over the legs. Inhale and return to starting position. Repeat 6 times and on the final time stay for a few breaths in the pose.

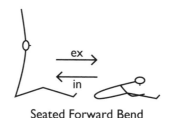

Seated Forward Bend

### 4. Tortoise Pose (*Kurmasana*)

Sit tall, legs just over hip width apart, knees bent. Lower the torso into a forward bend. Slip both arms under the knees and behind you to rest on the lower back. Or, for an easier alternative, catch hold of the outside of the ankles. Stay for a few breaths, drawing your awareness inward, and if you wish, silently repeat this affirmation: *I find peace within.*

*To work more gently, skip this pose.*

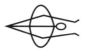

Tortoise Pose

## 5. Bridge Pose (*Setu Bandhasana*) with arm movements

Lie on your back, knees bent and hip width apart. Inhale and slowly peel the back from the floor and raise the arms above the head. Exhale and lower the back to the floor and simultaneously lower the arms. Repeat 6 times, staying for a few breaths the final time. Coordinate the breath with these phrases: *Open heart* (inhale) and *Blue-sky mind* (exhale).

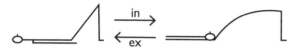

Bridge Pose with arm movements

## 6a. Bridge Pose (*Setu Bandhasana*)

Come into Bridge Pose as in step 5 but keep the arms by the sides. Clasp the hands under the body and stay in the pose for a few breaths. To ease the shoulders, just leave the arms by your sides, palms facing down.

## 6b. Bridge Pose (*Setu Bandhasana*) with leg raise

Come into Bridge Pose as in step 6a. Bend one knee into the chest and then straighten the leg, heel toward the ceiling. Stay for a few breaths. Do not allow the pelvis to tilt to one side. Repeat on the other side.

    *To work more gently, skip 6b.*

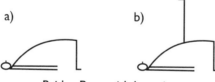

Bridge Pose with leg raise

## 7. Full-Body Stretch into Curl-Up

Inhale and lengthen tall along the floor. Exhale and bring the knees to the chest, curling the head and shoulders off the floor, and bring the hands to the knees. Inhale and return to Full-Body Stretch. Repeat 6 times.

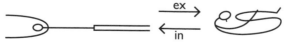

Full-Body Stretch into Curl-Up

## 8. Supine Twist (*Jathara Parivrtti*) modified

Bend both knees. For an easier pose, keep both feet on the floor. For more challenge, bring knees onto chest. Lay arms out to the side, just below shoulder height, palms facing downward. Exhale and lower both knees toward the floor on the left; turn head gently to the right. Inhale and come back to center. Repeat 6 times, alternating sides, and then stay in the pose for a few breaths on each side.

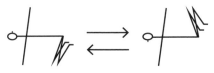

Supine Twist modified

## 9. Knees-to-Chest Pose (*Apanasana*)

Hug the knees into the chest and rest here for a few breaths.

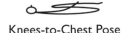

Knees-to-Chest Pose

## 10. Waterfall Breathing

This can be done sitting or lying down in the Relaxation Pose (*Savasana*). See *page 70* for instructions.

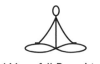

Waterfall Breathing

## Autumn Equinox Yoga Practice Overview

1. Mantra *Ma* and Arm Movements. Inhale: take arms out to the side. Exhale: bring hands back to the belly, chanting *Ma*. Stay for one breath with hands resting on belly. Repeat × 6.
2. *Ma-Om* Kneeling Sequence. Chanting *Ma,* come into Child's Pose from tall kneeling. Chanting *Om,* sit back into Child's Pose from all fours. Repeat × 4–6.
3. Seated Forward Bend. Inhale: raise both arms. Exhale: fold forward. Inhale: return to starting position. Repeat × 6, staying for a few breaths the final time.

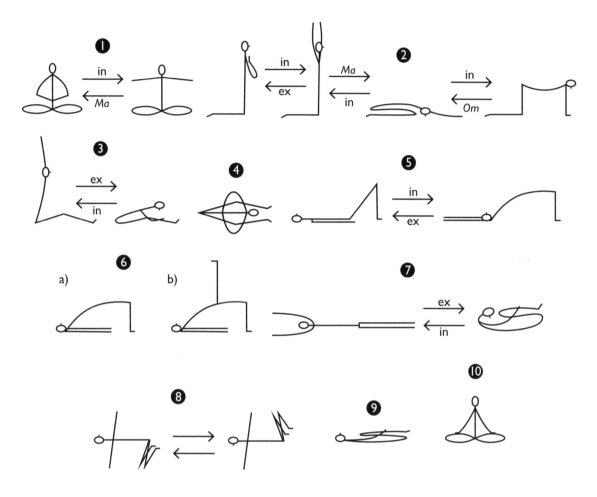

4. Tortoise Pose. Affirmation: *I find peace within.* Stay here for a few breaths, drawing your awareness inward. *Skip this pose for a gentler sequence.*

5. Bridge Pose with arm movements. Inhale: *Open heart.* Exhale: *Blue-sky mind.* Repeat × 6, staying for a few breaths the final time.

6a. Bridge Pose. Clasp hands under body and stay for a few breaths.

6b. Bridge Pose with leg raise. Stay for a few breaths. Repeat on other side.

7. Full-Body Stretch into Curl-Up. Inhale: lengthen tall along floor. Exhale: curl up. Repeat × 6.

8. Modified Supine Twist. Exhale: lower both knees toward floor on left, turn head right. Inhale: come back to center. Repeat × 6, alternating sides, and then stay for a few breaths in each pose on each side.

9. Knees-to-Chest Pose. Rest for a few breaths.

10. Waterfall Breathing.

---
### EXERCISE
## Waterfall Breathing

At the summer solstice waterfall breathing provides a watery counterbalance to the fiery, frenetic energy of the season. It can also be used at any other time of year.

*Waterfall breathing*, or the *divided out-breath*, can be used to calm a restless, agitated mind, inducing a state of deep calm and peacefulness. It soothes anxiety and dispels panic. It helps promote a good night's sleep.

If you prefer, this breathing practice can be used without using the waterfall imagery and will still be deeply relaxing.

Once you are familiar with the practice, you can do a shortened version, anywhere, anytime, over a few breaths. For the version below, allow about 10 minutes.

Find yourself a comfortable sitting position, spine tall and erect, shoulders relaxed down away from your ears. Soften your facial muscles with a half-smile.

Bring your awareness to your breathing. You do not need to control the breath. Just allow the breath to establish its own natural rhythm. Now become aware of and focus more on your exhale. Over several breaths begin to gently lengthen the exhale. Never strain with the breathing.

If it feels comfortable, begin to divide each exhale into two equal parts, with a pause in between each part. It looks like this:

> *Inhale*
> *Exhale, pause, exhale, and pause.*
> *Inhale…*

Imagine that with each part of the divided out-breath you are stepping down a step and then briefly pausing before stepping down another step.

If this feels comfortable, you can then go on to divide the out-breath into three equal parts, with pauses in between each part.

Now, for the time being, let go of dividing the breath and go back to your normal breathing.

Imagine that you are in a beautiful, peaceful place watching a gently cascading waterfall. Picture the water flowing down steps of rock into a calm pool below.

Keep this image of the cascading waterfall in your mind as you return again to the divided out-breath. Imagine that each part your out-breath is like water flowing down a waterfall and onto a ledge, where you pause briefly, and then exhale again, each part flowing down onto another ledge, before finally reaching a peaceful pool, where you pause briefly and then inhale. Repeat over several breaths.

When you feel ready, let go of the divided out-breath and the image of the waterfall. Simply observe the natural flow of the breath for a few more breaths.

Now let go of following the breath. Become aware of where your body is in contact with the floor or your support. Notice how you are feeling and observe how the waterfall breathing has affected you.[16] Resolve to take this calm, peaceful, open, and spacious awareness with you into your everyday life and the next thing that you do today.

## Tree Wisdom in Summer

Spending time around trees in summer connects us to the fertility and fullness of the season.

Summer is the perfect time to take a walk through the woods, forest, or park and enjoy the shade that trees provide. What effect does being amongst the trees have on your mood? Use all five senses to mindfully enjoy the scene; notice colors, smells, sounds and use your sense of touch. You might even find some edible forest fruit to take home and taste. Be aware of the diversity of life in the forest that trees support, such as insects, animals, and birds. Later, during a few quiet moments, close your eyes and recall this scene and enjoy a few moments of tranquility remembering this special environment.

---

16. Donna Farhi, *Yoga Mind, Body and Spirit: A Return to Wholeness* (New York, Henry Holt & Company, 2000), 250. Farhi uses waterfall imagery in her description of the Pacifying Breath.

# Trees and Creativity during Summer

You can use the time that you have spent mindfully amongst trees as a springboard for your creativity. If you are stuck for ideas, here are a few to get you going:

- Find a leaf that you find interesting because of its shape, color, texture, and so on. Then spend some time looking closely at it, and then draw it, either from observation or from memory.
- Make a list of five reasons why you feel grateful to trees.
- The breath is a key component of yoga. How much do you know about how trees breathe? Use the resources available to you online, in books, from a knowledgeable friend, and so on to find out more. Once you have done this, observe whether your newfound knowledge adds or detracts from your enjoyment and appreciation of trees.
- Compose a short guided visualization inspired by your walk in the forest. Make a recording of yourself reading this visualization and use it during a period of relaxation. If you have children, they might want to help you with this project. The recording you make can be relaxing for both of you.

## Meditation upon an Oak Tree at Summer Solstice

Near where I live is a grand stately home surrounded by acres of parkland, open to the public. The area is a site of special scientific interest because of its ancient oak trees. Deer graze and wildflowers grow around the trees; on the horizon you can see the silhouette of the Welsh hills.

We can learn from the oak tree about the strength and generosity contained within the circle of life, death, rebirth, and renewal. Below is the tree prose poem that I wrote in response to meditatively spending time around oak trees.

*Ancient oak tree, you connect me to the strength and courage to be found within me. From you I learn how to weather life's storms with grace. An acorn nestled in the soil, from small beginnings you grew into a mighty oak tree. Today, sunshine streaming through your crown creates a thousand emeralds of your leaves. Around your silver-gray trunk*

*grow golden buttercup, purple clover, and pink vetch. Swallows fly over-
head. The fragrance of orange blossom is carried on the breeze.*

*Oak tree, across the century, you have given sanctuary to insect,
animal, and bird. In your warm, fissured trunk insects make
their home. In your high branches birds build their nests. Wild deer
take refuge in your velvet shade. Caterpillars feast upon your leaves
and purple butterflies flit above your canopy. As you breathe out,
you breathe life into me. My inspiration is your generosity.*

## Summer Solstice Meditation Questions

These questions are designed to be used around the time of the summer solstice. It's fine to use them a week or two before or after the actual date of the solstice. Guidance on how to use the seasonal meditation questions can be found in chapter 1.

- Who brings sunshine into my life and how do I show my gratitude to them for this?
  - Who lights my fire and who am I passionate about?
  - How will I go about spending time with them this summer?

- Looking back over the past half year, what have I achieved? (This might include achievements at work, home, or study).
  - What has gone well and has come to fruition? How will I celebrate my success?
  - Which seeds failed to germinate and how would I do things differently next time to ensure success?
  - Who has helped me realize my dreams and how will I thank them?

- Where is the fiery passion in my life?
  - Over the past half year have I found time for doing the things I love to do?
  - What is on my love-to-do list for the remaining summer months?

- Summer solstice is a time associated with motherhood and fertility.
    - ↬ What was my own experience of being mothered/parented?
    - ↬ How would I be acting if I were to be a good mother/parent to myself?
    - ↬ (If you are a parent) How do I strengthen the bond between myself and my child (or grown-up child) in a supportive, loving, and healing way?

- At this fertile time, what am I creating in my life?
    - ↬ How do I nurture, nourish, and tend my creativity and my creations?
    - ↬ What blocks my creativity and how can I get my creativity flowing again?
    - ↬ How do I celebrate and enjoy my body and its natural rhythms in a loving and healthful way?

- At the summer solstice there is a gradual shift in energy from outward action to inner reflection and contemplation.
    - ↬ Which outward actions do I wish to bring inside to my inner sanctuary to be processed and transformed?
    - ↬ Do I value both my inner and outer worlds in equal measure?
    - ↬ Which seeds do I wish to incubate during the darker half of the year?
    - ↬ What do I want to nurture and develop in myself over the coming months?

- Following the summer solstice, the days will gradually begin to get shorter. How do I feel about moving into the darker half of the year?
    - ↬ How do I balance light and dark in myself?
    - ↬ How do I celebrate the return of the darkness? What value is there to be found in darkness?

- How will I go about bringing warmth and sunshine into the lives of friends, family, and the various communities that I am a part of?
    - ↬ How will I go about connecting with others this summer?
    - ↬ How can I lovingly shine my light out into the world?

• Are there any actions, big or small, that I can take this summer to make my neighborhood and immediate surroundings more beautiful, welcoming, or environmentally friendly?

• How do I plan to get out in nature and enjoy the beauty of the season?

CHAPTER FIVE

# Summer Turns to Autumn

*End of July to mid-September in the Northern Hemisphere*
*End of January to mid-March in the Southern Hemisphere*

This is the time of first harvest; apples are ripening on the tree and the corn is being brought in from the field. During the season of harvest, we take time to enjoy the cornucopian feast that nature has laid out before us. Whether we live in the city or the country, we can mindfully use our five senses to appreciate the bountifulness and abundance of the season.

## We Celebrate Summer's Abundance

Although it is high summer, autumn is visible on the horizon. The sun is gradually waning and losing its power: the days are getting shorter, and each morning the sun gets up a little later and goes to bed a little earlier. The energy of the earth is moving from fire to water, yang to yin, outer to inner, sun to moon, and if we can flow with this change of energy and gradually shift from outward pursuits to a more inward focus of contemplation, then it can be a wonderful way of keeping our life in balance.

Whether we are gardeners or not, we all have a harvest, and now is a good time to consider what you are harvesting. Look back over the past year and consider where you have been putting your energy and whether this has been fruitful or not. Your harvest may be the fruition of a project that is dear to your heart. Or perhaps it is the blossoming of a relationship that you have been nurturing. It might be the peacefulness that you have felt since you have established a regular yoga practice. Or perhaps it is literally vegetables and fruit that you've grown in your garden. Now is the time to honor your effort and celebrate what you have achieved.

The reaping of the harvest is associated with the theme of sacrifice. The grain harvest, in its passage from sheaf of corn to loaf of bread, is threshed, sifted, grounded, kneaded, and then assigned to the "sacred fire." In many traditions there are variations on the story of the God of Fire and Light being sacrificed to Mother Harvest. This is a good time to consider what needs to be sacrificed to ensure the success of your harvest. Sometimes to say yes to your passion, you must say no to something else that is less important to you.

Although the days are still warm and summery, the nights are gradually drawing in. We too draw our outward achievements inside, sorting the wheat from the chaff. The Sanskrit word for seed is *bija*. Contained within the harvest are the seeds of next year's crop. When you hold a grain of wheat or an apple pip in the palm of your hand, you are holding a miracle that is full of the potential for future growth.

What do you wish to preserve from your harvest? What are the seeds that you wish to store over the autumn and winter, ready for planting out next spring? The autumn and winter aren't the best time for action, but they are the perfect time to dream and make plans about what you wish to make manifest during next year's growing season. At harvest we draw our awareness back inside to the magical core at the heart of our being. We take our outer achievements inside to this wise, knowing, loving center at our core, to process them.

## Loving the Harvest and Harvesting Love

What will you give away with love this harvest season? Paradoxically, it is when we are sharing our wealth and giving it away that we feel most enriched. One way to celebrate abundance is to mindfully prepare a meal to share with your loved ones. As you prepare the food notice the colors of the ingredients, the smells, textures, and tastes. Remember not to forget the magic ingredient: love! Or you could make a harvest loaf plaited into a sheaf of wheat and share it with friends. Baking bread is a wonderful way of getting in touch with the harvest. Kneading the dough by hand is therapeutic and a great stress reliever too.

During the period of first harvest, we remember to say thank you to Mother Earth, as without her there is no harvest. One way of thanking the earth is to treat her with kindness and respect by embodying the yogic principle of non-harm or non-violence (*ahimsa*). We do this by considering what impact our actions are having upon the environment and aiming to act in a way that does the least harm. Some yogis choose to be vegetarian, others vegan, and some just cut down on meat and eat more vegetarian meals. If we all make some small changes to the way we live, then environmentally it will add up to a big difference. For example, at harvest you can reduce the air miles of food by buying delicious, fresh local produce. Or you can reduce air pollution, and improve fitness, by one day a week leaving the car at home. Your mantra: *Change begins with me*.

Another way to thank the earth is to simply notice the bounty and beauty that she spreads before us at harvest. We can get so caught up in the minutiae and busyness of our lives that we forget to look around us and appreciate the beauty of the season. To counteract this tendency, when you encounter something beautiful, stop and take time to enjoy it. Instead of habitually getting your phone out to capture the image digitally, occasionally just allow yourself the space to look and absorb the image into your mind's eye. Then when you are on your yoga mat, you can recall that beautiful flower, mountain view, dappled light in a forest, wheat field dancing in the breeze, or apples ripening on a tree, and let the image uplift you as you do your yoga. It will also help you strengthen your connection to the world around you. Yoga is union.

Traditionally, this is a time for festivals and community gatherings. Seek out others who share your love of yoga, and look for ways that you can share yoga's gifts with each other. Arrange a walking meditation in the park or a Sunday morning yoga session, followed by a shared picnic lunch. Be a force for good in your community. Look out for those small ways that you can improve the lives of your family, friends, colleagues, and wider community. Widen your circle of love. Karma yogis believe that what goes around comes around, so when you warm up your relationships, everyone benefits—including you!

Do you define an advanced yogi as someone who can tie themselves into pretzel-like shapes? Or is an advanced yogi someone who is kind to themselves and others? Perhaps you like the idea of doing a headstand or amazing your friends by doing a gravity-defying yoga balancing pose, whereas being kind to yourself and others sounds … well, a bit wimpy! However, steering yourself continually in the direction of kindness to yourself and others is anything but a soft option and is in fact spiritual warrior work. The Dalai Lama, when asked to sum up his spiritual practice, answered with two words: "Be kind."

Love is the harvest of your spiritual practice: we give out and gather in love. In the end your yoga practice will not be judged by how good you look in Lycra or by how long you can stay in a headstand or how many rounds of Salute to the Sun you can do. No, your spiritual practice will be judged by how much love you generated on and off the mat. And it is all those small acts of everyday kindness that add up to a life well lived. Love is the sweetest fruit of all.

## Harvesting Happiness, Gratitude, and Contentment

The Summer to Autumn Yoga Practice that follows this section focuses on cultivating contentment, gratitude, and happiness. Yoga Sutra 2.42 states, "Perfect happiness is attained through contentment."[17] When we cultivate gratitude as a spiritual practice, contentment (*samtosa*) naturally follows, and from contentment happiness blooms. Whereas happiness can be elusive, the path of gratitude and contentment is always available to us.

The season of first harvest is the perfect time to establish a gratitude practice. It is well documented that cultivating an attitude of gratitude has many health benefits, and research shows that gratitude improves our relationships: people who practice gratitude are more committed and responsive to their partners and are better listeners.[18]

One way that we can cultivate gratitude is by acknowledging all those people who have helped us "grow" our harvest. Saying thank you to someone who has helped you realize your harvest can be rewarding and fun. Take time to consider who has helped you and get creative, finding imaginative, fun ways of thanking them. Spread the love!

Part of our spiritual practice is to look deeply and to recognize that we are all part of an intricate web of interdependency. The self-made person is a myth. None of us can make it alone. Taking time to acknowledge with gratitude all the ways that we are supported by others is a spiritual act. It is important to recognize and show appreciation not just to our loved ones, but also to all those neutral people in our daily life. How do you treat that army of "invisible" people who provide you with services that enable your life

---

17. Barbara Stoler Miller, *Yoga: Discipline of Freedom; The Yoga Sutra of Patanjali* (New York: Bantam Books, 1998), 55.

18. Amie M. Gordon, "Gratitude Is for Lovers," *Greater Good Magazine*, February 5, 2013, https://greatergood.berkeley.edu/article/item/gratitude_is_for_lovers.

to run smoothly? Do you see and acknowledge the person who serves you in a restaurant and clears away after you? Do you remember to say thank you? Showing appreciation to all the supposedly "insignificant" people around us makes for a more civilized, humane society, and enriches our lives too. To strengthen your gratitude "muscle," try the Showing Appreciation Meditation, featured later in this chapter.

In our everyday life, by combining mindfulness with gratitude practice we are more able to relax into a contented state. Our mindfulness practice helps us pay attention to our experience as it unfolds, and our gratitude practice helps us savor, enjoy, and be thankful for all the little (and big) joys in our life as they arise from moment to moment.

Practicing gratitude before you go off to sleep helps you get a better night's sleep. Try counting off on your fingers ten things that you feel grateful for today. If you run out of things to be thankful for after the count of three, don't give up—keep going! It's important to get to ten so that you notice all those small blessings that you would normally take for granted, such as a mug of warm tea, a hot shower, the succulent taste of a juicy peach, a child's smile, or the sun on your face.

The contentment we find in our yoga practice energizes us to take the actions that will help us find happiness in our lives. Yoga postures, breathing, and relaxation induce states of calm and serenity; this in turn prepares the ground for meditation. With mind and body calm and at ease, during meditation we slip into a state of deep contentment. In this contented state we are neither pushed nor pulled by whatever arises; we neither grasp for happiness nor push away unhappiness; we allow things to be as they are. This meditative, contented state is truly a healthy, wholesome, healing place to be.

At harvest our yoga practice helps us draw inward and uncover within ourselves the beauty and potential that lies at our center. As the Earth spins its way around the wheel of the year, we stay connected to that kind, compassionate heart within. In this way we weather happiness and heartache, the gains and loss, and the ups and downs that the turning of the year brings us. Though the seasons may bring wind, rain, sunshine, or showers, we remain connected to ourselves, to each other, and to the earth.

## Summer to Autumn Yoga Practice

This yoga practice is inspired by the abundance of the first harvest, and it cultivates a sense of gratitude for the earth's abundance. Yoga Sutra 2.42 states, "Perfect happiness is attained through contentment." [19] We integrate Patanjali's words on contentment into the practice as a way of opening ourselves up to happiness.

As summer transitions to autumn, we move from outward activity to focusing on inner contemplation. This change is reflected in this yoga practice by combining opening yoga poses with closing ones (e.g., as in Warrior with open arms into Intense Side Stretch Pose in step 3 below).

The practice has been designed to be used from late summer through early autumn, although it's fine to use at any time of year. It's both energizing and calming and has a balancing (*samana*) effect. It uplifts and encourages a positive attitude.

Allow 15 to 30 minutes.

### 1. Cultivating Gratitude Exercise, standing

Stand tall, feet hip width apart. Name three things that you feel grateful for today.

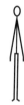

Cultivating Gratitude Exercise, standing

### 2. Albatross Sequence 1

Stand tall, feet hip width apart. Inhale and raise arms above head. Exhale and bend forward, about 45 degrees, back slightly arched, spreading arms out to the sides like a bird's wings (this is Albatross Pose). Stay for one breath in the pose. Inhale and come back up to standing, sweeping arms above head. Exhale and lower arms back to sides. Repeat the sequence 4 to 6 times.

---

19. Barbara Stoler Miller, *Yoga: Discipline of Freedom; The Yoga Sutra of Patanjali* (New York: Bantam Books, 1998), 55.

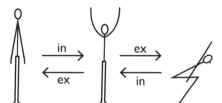

Albatross Sequence 1

## 3. Warrior Pose (*Virabhadrasana*) variation into
## Intense Side Stretch Pose (*Parsvottanasana*) variation

Stand tall, feet hip width apart, both hands resting on the belly. Step one foot forward. Inhale and take the arms out to the side and bend the front knee. Exhale and bend forward over the front leg, sweeping both arms behind the back. Inhale and come back up, sweeping the arms out to the side. Exhale and straighten the front leg and return the hands to the belly. Repeat 3 times and then repeat on the other side. As you inhale, silently say, *Perfect happiness*. As you exhale, *Contentment*.

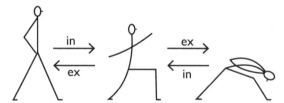

Warrior Pose variation into Intense Side Stretch Pose variation

## 4. Bow to the Earth (*Bhumi Pranam*)

Stand tall, feet hip width apart, hands in Prayer Pose (*Namaste*). Stay here for a few breaths focusing on the heart chakra (*anahata*). Keeping hands together, raise arms above the head; stay here a few breaths, focusing on the space above the crown of the head, the crown chakra (*sahasrara*). Lower the prayer hands to the third eye chakra (*ajna*) and then the throat chakra (*vishuddha*). Bend the knees deeply (thighs parallel to the floor) and bring the prayer hands to touch the floor. Stay here for a few breaths, silently repeating, "I thank the earth for supporting me." Inhale and come back up to standing, taking prayer hands above the head. Exhale and lower prayer hands back to heart. Repeat 3 times.

*If you are short of time, finish your practice finish here.*

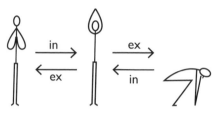

Bow to the Earth

### 5. Lunge Pose (*Anjaneyasana*) with arm movements

Come to tall kneeling. Take your right foot forward; bend the knee, bringing the knee over the ankle. Rest your fingertips lightly on your ears, elbows out to the side. Exhale and round the back forward, looking down. Inhale and open up the chest, pull the elbows back, and look up slightly. Repeat 4 times and then stay in the open chest position for a few breaths. Repeat on the other side.

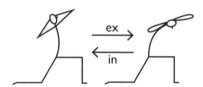

Lunge Pose with arm movements

### 6. Downward-Facing Dog Pose (*Adho Mukha Svanasana*)

Come onto all fours; turn the toes under and push up into Downward-Facing Dog Pose. Stay here for a few breaths.

Downward-Facing Dog Pose

### 7. Half-Locust Pose (*Ardha Salabhasana*)

Lie on your front, head facing down and arms by your sides. Inhale to prepare. Exhale and raise the upper body in to a backbend, sweeping the arms out to the side like a bird's wings, and at the same time lift one straight leg from the floor. (Keep both frontal pelvic bones on the floor; do not twist the pelvis as you come into the backbend.) Inhale and lift the chest a little higher. Exhale and lower to the starting position. Repeat on the other side. Repeat 4 times each side, alternating sides.

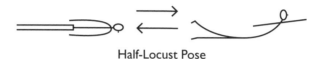

Half-Locust Pose

### 8. Locust Pose (*Salabhasana*)

Lie on your front, head facing down and arms by your sides. Inhale to prepare. Exhale and come up into a backbend, and at the same time raise both straight legs from the floor (keep both frontal pelvic bones on the floor; do not twist the pelvis as you come into the backbend); arms stay by your sides. Inhale and lift the chest a little higher. Exhale and lower back down to the starting position. Repeat 4 times and on the final time stay for a few breaths in the pose.

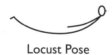

Locust Pose

### 9. Cat Pose (*Marjaryasana*) into Child's Pose (*Balasana*)

Come onto all fours. Exhale and lower the bottom to the heels and the head to the floor to Child's Pose (*Balasana*). Inhale and come back up to all fours. Repeat 6 times. As you inhale, silently say, *Perfect happiness*. As you exhale, *Contentment*.

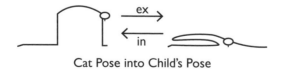

Cat Pose into Child's Pose

### 10a. Supine Twist (*Jathara Parivrtti*)

Lie on your back, knees bent, feet together, arms out to the sides at shoulder height, palms facing down. Bring both knees onto your chest. Exhale and lower both knees down toward the floor on the left. Inhale and return to center. Repeat 6 times each side, alternating sides.

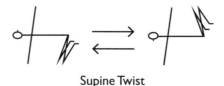

Supine Twist

### 10b. Supine Twist (*Jathara Parivrtti*) variation

Then drop your knees to the left; place your left hand on the top of your right thigh, gently persuading your legs down toward the floor. Turn your right palm up and, keeping your arm in contact with the floor, raise your arm up toward your right ear. Stay here for a few breaths. And then repeat on the other side.

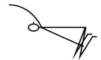

Supine Twist variation

### 11. Knees-to-Chest Pose (*Apanasana*) into Leg Raises

Bring both knees onto your chest. Inhale and straighten your legs to the vertical, heels toward the ceiling; taking your arms out to the side, just below shoulder height, palms facing up. Exhale and bring knees back to chest (*Apanasana*). Repeat 6 times.

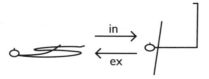

Knees-to-Chest Pose into Leg Raises

## 12. The Showing Appreciation Meditation

See page 88.

The Showing Appreciation Meditation

## Summer to Autumn Yoga Practice Overview

1. Cultivating Gratitude Exercise, standing. Name three things you are grateful for today.

2. Albatross Sequence 1. Repeat × 4–6.

3. Warrior variation into Intense Side Stretch Pose variation. Inhale: *Perfect happiness.* Exhale: *Contentment.* Repeat × 3 and then repeat on other side.

4. Bow to the Earth. Say, *I thank the earth for supporting me.* Repeat × 3.

5. Lunge Pose with arm movements. Repeat × 4 and then stay in open chest position for a few breaths. Repeat on other side.

6. Downward-Facing Dog Pose. Stay for a few breaths.

7. Half-Locust Pose. Repeat × 4 on each side, alternating sides.

8. Locust Pose. Repeat × 4 and on final time stay for a few breaths.

9. Cat Pose into Child's Pose. Inhale: *Perfect happiness.* Exhale: *Contentment.* Repeat × 6.

10a. Supine Twist. Repeat × 6, alternating sides.

10b. Stay here for a few breaths. Repeat on other side.

11. Knees-to-Chest Pose into Leg Raises. Repeat × 6.

12. The Showing Appreciation Meditation.

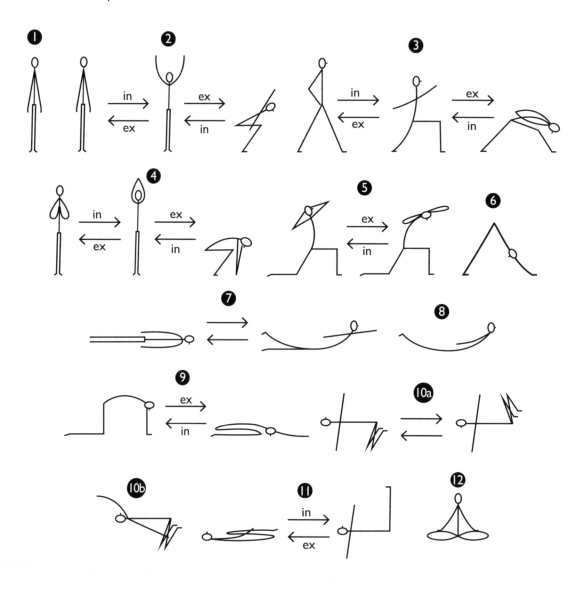

## EXERCISE

# The Showing Appreciation Meditation

This meditation can be done any time of year, although it is particularly appropriate during the harvest season, as a way of cultivating gratitude toward all those people (including ourselves!) who have helped us realize our harvest and made life run more smoothly. It helps strengthen our gratitude "muscle" and stops us from taking people for granted. It engenders positive feelings toward ourselves and others.

Allow 10 to 20 minutes.

Find yourself a comfortable but erect sitting position, either on the floor or in an upright chair. Or, if you prefer, this meditation can be done lying down.

Relax the parts of your body that are in contact with the floor, or your support, down into the earth.

Let go of any unnecessary tension, relax your shoulders down away from your ears, and soften your face by adopting a half smile.

Now become aware of the natural flow of your breath and maintain a background awareness of the breath throughout the meditation.

We begin by cultivating a sense of gratitude and loving kindness toward ourselves. Recall three things that make you feel grateful toward yourself. If you are finding it hard to think of anything, see if you can find just one small thing you like about yourself and feel grateful for. If you find yourself lapsing into self-criticism, congratulate yourself for noticing this and send yourself some love and compassion.

Now silently repeat several times the loving kindness phrases for yourself:

> *May I be safe.*
> *May I be happy.*
> *May I be healthy.*
> *May I live with ease.*

Now bring to mind someone whom you are close to and who helps your life to run more smoothly. Consider all the things that this person does for you, big or small, and all the ways that they improve your quality of life. Send your gratitude and thanks to this person; thank them for the many ways they contribute to your happiness.

If you are finding it hard today to think of anyone, you could remember someone who has helped you and supported you in the past. Or, if it is easier, send good wishes to a pet who brings joy into your life.

Now silently repeat the loving kindness phrases a few times for this person (if you wish, you can insert their name into the phrase):

> *May you be safe.*
> *May you be happy.*
> *May you be healthy.*
> *May you live with ease.*

Now bring to mind a neutral person, someone who helps you in some way but who you don't know very well. Choose someone who you don't have strong feelings toward either way, but who makes your life run more smoothly. Perhaps they are someone who delivers your mail or serves you in a shop, a cleaner at your place of work, or a bus driver. Send your gratitude and thanks to this person; thank them for the help that they give to you. Silently repeat the loving kindness phrases a few times for this person:

> *May you be safe.*
> *May you be happy.*
> *May you be healthy.*
> *May you live with ease.*

Now picture yourself, your friend, and the neutral person all together. Picture all three of you looking safe, happy, healthy, and at ease. Just like you, the friend and the neutral person want to be happy and free from suffering. Just like you, their lives have ups and downs. And just like you, they rely on others to help and support them and to make their life run smoothly.

Repeat the loving kindness phrases for the three of you:

> *May we all be safe.*
> *May we all be happy.*
> *May we all be healthy.*
> *May we all live with ease.*

After repeating the phrases a number of times, let them go and finish by once more sending yourself good wishes, loving kindness, and compassion.

Now bring your awareness back to the sensations associated with where your body is in contact with the floor or your support. Become aware of the natural rhythm of your breath again. Notice how you are feeling and be aware of any insights that you've gained from doing this meditation. Become aware of your surroundings. Have a good stretch and do any movements you need to do to wake the body up.

Resolve to take these feelings of love, kindness, and gratitude for yourself and others back into your everyday life.

## Tree Wisdom: Summer to Autumn

Spending time around trees is the perfect way to connect to the abundance of the season of first fruits and harvest. When you're out walking, look out for the signs of the fruitfulness of trees: acorns forming on oak trees, conkers on horse chestnut trees, berries on the hawthorn tree, and, of course, fruit on fruit trees. Mindfully observe a tree that you feel drawn to with an open mind and curiosity. Use your five senses to enjoy and appreciate its fruitfulness.

### EXERCISE
# Trees and Creativity during Summer to Autumn

You can use the time that you have spent mindfully around trees as a springboard for your creativity. If you are stuck for ideas, here are a few to get you going:

- Take photos of the fruit and seeds that you observe on trees. Make a collage of them and post it on your favorite social media site. Or use the collage as a screen saver.
- Find a fruit from a tree, such as a conker, acorn, berry, or other fruit, and use it to inspire you to mindfully write a poem, compose a song, paint a picture, or make a collage out of objects found in nature. (If you have kids, they may want to join in this activity!)
- How much do you know about the science of how trees reproduce? Use the resources available to you online, in books, from a knowledgeable friend,

and so on to find out more. Once you have done this, observe whether your newfound knowledge adds to or detracts from your enjoyment and appreciation of trees. Share your knowledge with friends.

- Mindfully cook something with fruits that you have grown or found growing wild (only eat wild food if you are certain it is edible) or buy some seasonal fruit from your local shop.
- Try out the Apple Mindfulness Meditation in this chapter.

## Meditation upon a Crab Apple Tree at Harvest

Last August I was walking in the countryside with my husband. We were both feeling low because his elderly mum had recently died, and we had been talking about where to scatter her ashes. As we passed through a wooden gate leading from a field into the woods, I noticed a wild crab apple tree laden with apples, its branches intertwined with an oak tree. We stood and admired the beauty of the trees for a few moments and somehow it lifted our spirits. Below is the tree prose poem that I wrote in response to meditatively spending time around this crab apple tree.

> *Your path leads you through a grove of trees. Two white butterflies zigzag playfully and draw your gaze to the branches of a crab apple tree, linked arm in arm with an oak. Shafts of rainbow-sunlight filter through the trees and do a dance of sunlight and shadow upon the woodland floor, which is carpeted with blackberries ripening on the brambles, pink campion, and yellow daisies. Beyond the trees a field of golden grain is bathed in sunshine. Swallows fly overhead, and white clouds drift across blue sky to the mountains.*

> *The crab apple tree gives pollen and nectar to the bees; blackbirds and thrushes eat her apples and disperse the seed. She is laden down with love, her branches heavy with apples and the seeds of possibility.*
> *The Apple-Mother takes all your cares and woes and scatters them like apple blossom on the wind. The seeds of love bear fruit, she says, give all your love away. Give all your love away today, your love will be returned to you, give all your love away.*

---
EXERCISE
---
# Apple Mindfulness Meditation

You will need an apple and a kitchen knife. Allow 5 to 10 minutes.

Sit on an upright chair at a table. Place your apple on the table in front of you.

Imagine that you have never seen an apple before. Look at the apple; notice its shape, its color, its texture; notice where it catches the light and where it is in shade.

Now pick the apple up and hold it in your hands. Explore the apple with your hands; enjoy its shape, its curves, and its texture. Notice its color and how it catches the light.

Now place the apple on the table again. Pick up your knife and, with care, cut transversely across the middle of the apple. Replace your knife back on the table. Smell the sweetness of the cut apple. Hold the two halves of apple in your hands: What do you see? If you look closely, you will notice that hidden inside the apple is a five-pointed star in a circle around the core. It looks like a flower with five petals contained within the circle of the apple.

Now remove one pip from the apple's core. Cradle the pip in the palm of your hand, noticing its shape, color, and how it catches the light. Take the pip between your thumb and first finger; roll it about to feel its texture. Notice how although the pip is so small, at the same time it contains within it the potential of a future apple tree.

When you are ready, slowly and mindfully eat your apple, enjoying and savoring each mouthful.

## Summer to Autumn Meditation Questions

These questions are designed to be used any time from around the end of July to mid-August in the Northern Hemisphere and from around the end of January to mid-February in the Southern Hemisphere. Guidance on how to use the seasonal meditation questions can be found in chapter 1.

- This is the season of harvest. What is my own personal harvest?
    - ⤙ Who has helped me realize my harvest and how will I thank them?
    - ⤙ How will I celebrate my harvest and how will I share my abundance with others?

- What are the seeds inherent in my harvest?
  - ↪ Which seeds will I be incubating over the autumn-to-winter season, ready to plant out next spring?
  - ↪ Which of my outer achievements need to be taken inside to be processed, the wheat sorted from the chaff?

- What do I need to sacrifice in order to realize my harvest? What needs weeding out or cutting back to ensure the success of my harvest?
  - ↪ Do I use my time wisely and are there any activities that I could drop in order to ensure that what really matters to me is fruitful?

- What am I harvesting in my personal relationships?
  - ↪ Which relationships have been fruitful and how will I celebrate them?
  - ↪ Where relationships have not been fruitful, do I need to invest more time and energy in them or do I need to let them go?
  - ↪ How can I help those close to me realize their potential so that they might lead fruitful and fulfilling lives?
  - ↪ How will I go about spending time with my loved ones over the remaining weeks of summer, and what can we do together that would bring us closer and give us both pleasure?

- What am I grateful for in my life?
  - ↪ Do I regularly notice and savor all my everyday blessings?
  - ↪ Am I able to acknowledge suffering in both my own life and other people's lives while at the same time still appreciate and enjoy the beauty of life?

- What am I harvesting in my yoga practice?
  - ↪ Have I put in the time and energy required to ensure a fruitful practice?
  - ↪ What are the strengths of my practice and how could I build on these?
  - ↪ What do I love about yoga and how can I share this love with others?

• The earth is so bountiful giving us the harvest. What small steps could I take this season to give back to the earth and to ensure that she continues to flourish?

• How will I go about connecting with nature and enjoying with all my senses the fruitfulness and beauty of the season?

CHAPTER SIX

# Autumn Equinox

*September 20–23 in the Northern Hemisphere*
*March 20–23 in the Southern Hemisphere*

The autumn equinox is the perfect time to explore balance in your yoga practice. And yoga is the perfect way to bring balance to body and mind.

## The Wisdom of Autumn

At the autumn equinox night and day are balanced before we tip in to the darkest phase of the year. The dark will continue to expand until the sun is reborn at the winter solstice in December, when the light phase of the year begins anew.

*Equinox* is derived from Latin and means "equal night." At both equinoxes Earth is perfectly balanced, with its North and South Poles tilted neither toward nor away from the sun, making day and night equal all over the world.

At the autumn equinox there is a shift of emphasis from sun to moon, light to dark, action to contemplation, growth to dormancy, fruitfulness to composting, building up to letting go, and movement to stillness. Now is a good time to pause after the frenetic activity of the growing season and consider how best to recuperate, regenerate, and replenish your energy this autumn.

This is the season of the final harvest and a good time to get together with others to celebrate and share the bounty of the earth. At my autumn yoga days, I ask participants to bring along something from their own personal harvest to donate to a harvest table. The idea is to donate something and take something else away at the end of the day. It's wonderful to see the table heaving with produce, a biscuit tin brim-full of slices of homemade apple cake, bags bursting with apples, containers of garden-grown grapes, paper bags stuffed with runner beans, a huge marrow, and jars of jam and chutneys.

In autumn there is poignancy in the misty, mellow fruitfulness of the season, combined with a wistful longing that summer might never end. However, once we let go of summer and accept the arrival of autumn, it is a time rich with possibilities.

Nature responds to diminishing hours of daylight by gradually withdrawing into dormancy; leaves fall from the trees, vegetation dies back, and some animals prepare to hibernate. We too can honor our connection to nature and respond with wisdom to the changing season by changing our focus from activity and outward action to contemplation and inner reflection. This process of drawing inward is a continuation of the work begun at the summer solstice, when the sun's powers began to wane and we entered the darker half of the year. In yoga we have the concept of *pratyahara,* which is a withdrawing of the senses from external stimuli. We are approaching a time for simply being and dreaming up plans for next year's growing season.

## Balanced Planet and Balanced You

Twice a year at the equinoxes our planet returns to a neutral, balanced state. As yoga practitioners, we can learn the art of balance by observing the earth's graceful seasonal cycle of balance, activity, balance, rest. In our yoga practice, we too can create a healing space by learning to recognize and return to this neutral, balanced state. This state of equanimity and equilibrium is our home base, giving our body, mind, and emotions the space to realign and heal.

During our yoga practice, we move in and out of this neutral, balanced state. We begin each yoga session by pausing to find neutral, and in this way we come home to ourselves. During the pause, we recognize tension in our body, make subtle adjustments to our posture, observe the torrent of thoughts passing through the mind, tune in to our natural breath, and let things settle. This pause provides a transition from our everyday life and activities into the sacred space of yoga. Then during our yoga practice, between more dynamic postures, we return to neutral in *asanas* such as Mountain Pose (*Tadasana*), Easy Pose (*Sukhasana*), or Relaxation Pose (*Savasana*). And then at the end of the practice we conclude by coming back to neutral, and this makes for a smooth transition between our yoga practice and getting back to everyday life.

In neutral our body's inherent wisdom is revealed, and it instinctively knows how to readjust and correct itself. Yoga teaches us to recognize neutral, both on a gross level in our body and on the subtler psychic and spiritual plane. In the stillness of this neutral state, we can hear and respond to the still, small voice of calm within.

The skill that we learn on the yoga mat of returning to this neutral, balanced state can also be applied to everyday life. How does it feel when your life is in balance? How is it different from when your life is out of balance?

We create balance in our lives by being clear about what and who are important to us. This enables us to defend our energy from being hijacked by things that are trivial and don't really matter to us. This clarity gives us the confidence to say "yes!" to the things that we value and to be comfortable saying "no!" to that which is depleting and takes us away from the life we want to live.

A strong network of family and friends provides us with the stability and grounding we need to walk the tightrope of life. If we take a wrong step and fall, they are our safety net. They alert us to when we have strayed off balance. Strong, supportive connections with our community, family, and friends help us feel stable and rooted. We learn to give and to accept support, to be there for others, and in our hour of need we hope they will be there for us too.

When our life is out of balance, we feel cut off from the flow of life. We don't feel at home in our own skin. We are somewhere else, not in the present. We feel time pressured, unable to find time for doing the things that we love, the things that nourish us and bring us back to a balanced state.

When our life is in balance, we feel connected, carried by the flow of life, on the right track, happy, optimistic, generous, and tolerant of others. When balance is present in our life, there is enough time, things get done with ease, there is enough love, and we feel held by the web of life.

## Celebrating Harvest and the Autumn Art of Letting Go

If you are a gardener, you will have a tangible harvest: ripe tomatoes, huge marrows, green beans, colorful sweet peas, jars of apple chutney. Those of us who are not gardeners might find it harder to define our personal harvest. Take time to acknowledge, appreciate, and celebrate even your most subtle achievements. Look deeply and be prepared to sing your own praises. At the same time note which seeds failed to germinate, honestly evaluating and learning from any failures. Thank everyone who has helped you realize your harvest.

The nights are drawing in and we too draw our outer achievements inside for processing and composting. We retrieve the seeds inherent within our harvest, storing them, ready to plant out next spring. Although the dark phase of the year is not the best time for action, it's an excellent time to incubate ideas, strategize, plan, and dream. Then we will be perfectly placed to spring into action when next spring comes around again.

There is wisdom to be found in the fading beauty of autumn. In spring the newly formed leaf contains within itself the blueprint that prompts it to fall from the tree in autumn. The tree knows that to survive the dark, cold winter months it must conserve energy. Over winter, the fallen leaves rot, forming compost that in turn nourishes the tree. And when spring comes around, new buds unfurl into fresh green leaves.

By observing and responding to the changing seasons, our awareness of the cycle of life, death, and rebirth is heightened. When we combine this seasonal awareness with meditation, we find ourselves more able to embrace the cycle of life, death, and rebirth. We find peace in a world that is constantly changing.

The tree in autumn provides the inspiration for this chapter's Autumn Equinox Yoga Practice. We can imitate the wisdom of the tree by conserving energy over the coming autumn and winter months and letting go of unnecessary baggage. This process of letting go enables us to create a sense of physical and mental spaciousness in our lives. Letting go is about prioritizing what's important to us and clearing a space, both physical and psychic, to nurture and nourish the things that do matter to us. To help you to cultivate the art of letting go, our autumn yoga practice concludes with the Placing Thoughts on a Leaf Visualization.

During the autumn and winter months our focus is on the inner journey. We can find a route map for this journey by studying the last three of Patanjali's limbs of yoga, which are concentration (*dharana*), meditation (*dhyana*), and contemplation (*samadhi*). Meditation allows us to let go of mental clutter and creates a sense of blue-sky spaciousness.

## Autumn Equinox Yoga Practice

This practice uses visualization to help you to connect with nature and the changing season. As autumn arrives and the year winds down, nature takes steps to conserve energy and let go of that which is unnecessary; this practice will enable you to begin that same process of conserving energy and sensory withdrawal (*pratyahara*).

It also celebrates harvest and gives you the opportunity to consider which seeds you wish to incubate over the winter months, ready to send up green shoots next spring.

The practice is designed to be used around the time of the autumn equinox, but it's fine to use it at any time of year. It has a calming effect, enabling you to let go of everyday cares and preoccupations. It will help you ground and center yourself and has a balancing effect.

Allow 15 to 20 minutes.

### 1. Standing Like a Tree in Autumn

Stand tall, feet hip width apart. Picture a tree in all its autumn splendor.

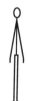

Standing Like a Tree in Autumn

### 2. Bend and Straighten Warm-Up

Take the feet just over hip width apart, toes turned slightly out, arms out to the side just below shoulder height. Exhale and bend both knees over the feet; lower the arms. Inhale and return to the starting position. Repeat 8 times.

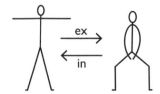

Bend and Straighten Warm-Up

### 3. Tree Pose (*Vrksasana*)

Stand tall, feet hip width apart; hands in Prayer Position (Namaste). Picture a tree in all its autumn splendor. Imagine that like a tree you have roots going from the soles of your feet way down into the earth. Then bring the sole of your right foot to rest on your inner left thigh, rotating your right knee out to the side. Either keep your hands at the heart or take your arms above the head, hands in prayer position. Fix your gaze on a point that is not moving. Stay for a few breaths. Repeat on the other side.

If you have balance problems, instead of bringing the foot onto the thigh, just rest the sole of the foot on the opposite inside ankle or be near a wall for support.

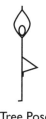

Tree Pose

### 4. Cat Pose (*Marjaryasana*) into Cow Pose (*Bitilasana*)

Start on all fours. Exhale and round the back up like an angry cat (*Marjaryasana*). Inhale into Cow Pose (*Bitilasana*), arching the back, lifting the chest up and away from the belly, and looking up slightly. Alternate between these two positions, rounding and arching the back. (If you have a back problem, don't arch the back.) Repeat 8 times.

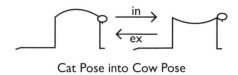

Cat Pose into Cow Pose

### 5. Child's Pose (*Balasana*) into
### Upward-Facing Dog (*Urdhva Mukha Svanasana*)

From Cow Pose (step 4) bend the knees and sit back into Child's Pose (*Balasana*), arms outstretched along the floor. From Child's Pose inhale and move forward into Upward-

Facing Dog (*Urdhva Mukha Svanasana*), arching your back and keeping your knees on the floor. Stay for one breath. Exhale back into Child's Pose. Repeat 6 times.

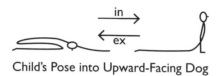

Child's Pose into Upward-Facing Dog

## 6. Seated Forward Bend (*Paschimottanasana*)

Sit tall, legs outstretched (bend the knees to ease the pose). Inhale and raise both arms. Exhale and fold forward over the legs. Inhale and return to starting position. Repeat 6 times. Then stay in the pose for a few breaths, and as you do so ask yourself this question: *In autumn, as the trees let go of their leaves, what do I wish to let go of?*

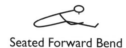

Seated Forward Bend

## 7. Supine Tree Pose (*Supine Vrksasana*)

Lie on your back, legs outstretched along the floor. Bring the sole of your left foot to rest on the inner right thigh; allow the right knee to rotate out to the side (to ease the pose, put a support under the knee). Take the arms above the head, bringing the fingertips lightly together (or to ease the pose, take the arms out at shoulder height, palms facing up). Stay here for a few breaths, picturing a tree in autumn. Repeat on the other side.

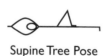

Supine Tree Pose

## 8. Full-Body Stretch into Curl-Up

Inhale and lengthen tall along the floor. Exhale and bring the knees to the chest, curling the head and shoulders off the floor, and bring the hands to the knees. Inhale and return to Full-Body Stretch. Repeat 4 times.

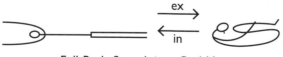

Full-Body Stretch into Curl-Up

### 9. Supine Butterfly Pose (*Supta Baddha Konasana*)

Lie on your back, knees spread out to the sides and soles of feet together; your hands can either rest on your belly or above your head. For comfort, prop your knees on bolsters, cushions, or blocks. Silently repeat this affirmation: *I welcome abundance into my life.*

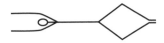

Supine Butterfly Pose

### 10. Full-Body Stretch

Take the arms above the head and lengthen tall along the floor.

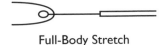

Full-Body Stretch

### 11. Knees-to-Chest Pose (*Apanasana*)

Hug the knees into the chest. Rest here for a few breaths, contemplating this question: What do I wish to incubate over the winter, ready to send up green shoots next spring?

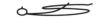

Knees-to-Chest Pose

### 12. Placing Thoughts on a Leaf Visualization

See page 106.

Placing Thoughts on a Leaf Visualization

### Autumn Equinox Yoga Practice Overview

1. Standing Like a Tree. Picture a tree in all its autumn splendor.
2. Bend and Straighten Warm-Up. Exhale: bend both knees and lower arms. Inhale: return to starting position. Repeat × 8.
3. Tree Pose. Picture a tree in autumn. Stay for a few breaths. Repeat on other side.

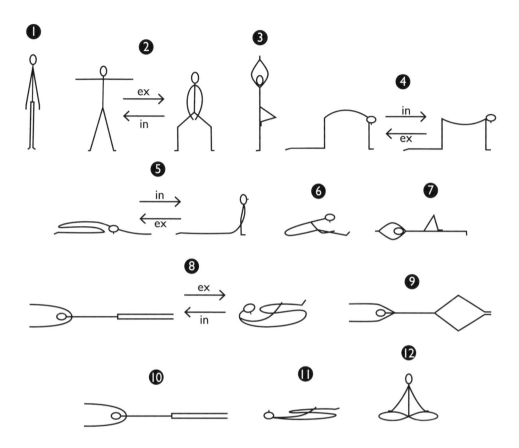

4. Cat Pose to Cow Pose. Repeat × 8.

5. Child's Pose into Upward-Facing Dog Pose. Inhale: move from Child's Pose into Upward-Facing Dog pose; stay one breath. Exhale: sit back into Child's Pose; stay one breath. Repeat × 6.

6. Seated Forward Bend. Ask: *In autumn, as the trees let go of their leaves, what do I wish to let go of?*

7. Supine Tree Pose. Stay for a few breaths, picturing a tree in autumn. Repeat on other side.

8. Full-Body Stretch into Curl-Up. Inhale: lengthen tall along the floor. Exhale: curl up. Inhale: return to stretch. Repeat × 4.

9. Supine Butterfly Pose. Affirmation: *I welcome abundance into my life.*

10. Full-Body Stretch. Lengthen tall along the floor.

11. Knees-to-Chest Pose. Ask: *What do I wish to incubate over the winter, ready to send up green shoots next spring?*

12. Placing Thoughts on a Leaf Visualization.

EXERCISE
## Placing Thoughts on a Leaf Visualization

The Placing Thoughts on a Leaf Visualization can be done at any time of year but is particularly good to do when the leaves are falling from the trees in autumn. It soothes a restless and agitated mind; it brings focus to the mind and quietens persistent, unwanted thoughts.[20]

It can be done sitting or lying down and takes about 10 minutes.

Find yourself a comfortable position either sitting or lying down. If you are sitting, establish an erect but relaxed posture.

Begin by noticing any thoughts and feelings that are passing through your mind. Simply observe thoughts and feelings without judgment as they come and go.

Now bring your awareness to sensations arising in your body. Notice which parts of your body already feel relaxed and where there is discomfort or tension.

Become aware of the natural flow of your breath. Notice how your belly rises and falls with each in- and out-breath. Throughout the meditation maintain a background awareness of the natural wavelike flow of your breath.

Now imagine that it is a sunny day and you are sitting under a tree on the riverbank, watching the river flow by. Shafts of sunlight stream through the trees and sparkle on the water below … The river is like a mirror reflecting blue sky, white clouds, and rippling trees. The wind whispers through the branches of the trees and blows autumn leaves onto the water below … You watch the leaves, noticing their different shapes and colors as they sail by …

---

20. This exercise uses "placing thoughts on a leaf" imagery from Susan M. Orsillo and Lizabeth Roemer, *The Mindful Way through Anxiety: Break Free from Chronic Anxiety and Reclaim Your Life* (New York: The Guilford Press, 2011), 184–85.

Now once again return your awareness to noticing thoughts as they come and go in your mind. Imagine that as a thought arises you place it onto a leaf and watch the leaf float by. And then when another thought comes into your mind, place that thought on a leaf too and watch it sail away downstream.

If your mind gets carried away by a torrent of thoughts and feelings, congratulate yourself for noticing this, and then simply begin again by placing the next thought that comes into your mind onto a leaf. If thoughts come into your mind that the meditation isn't working or that you're not doing it right, these are just thoughts, so just place them on a leaf too and watch them float by…

We're not trying to get rid of thoughts. You don't need to push thoughts away. We're simply observing the stream of thoughts passing through the mind and letting them float away in their own time.

Now let go of placing your thoughts on leaves. Widen your awareness to take in the whole of your imagined river scene. What do you see? Notice shapes, colors, and textures. What do you hear? Use your five senses to really picture the scene around you. Particularly, be aware of changes that herald the arrival of autumn. Enjoy the beauty of the place.

Now let go of picturing the river scene. Bring your awareness back to noticing sensations in your body and where your body is in contact with the floor or support. Notice how you are feeling now and how the meditation has affected you. Become aware of sounds inside the room and sounds outside the room. Become aware of your surroundings and when you are ready, open your eyes. Take this peaceful, patient, accepting, and more spacious awareness into the next activity you do today.

EXERCISE

# Sending Loving Kindness to the Earth Meditation

This meditation can be done any time of year, although it is particularly appropriate at harvest time as a way of showing gratitude for the earth's bounty. It is particularly apt for the equinoxes, as in the meditation we are picturing a world that has regained the balance of a healthy ecosystem.

This meditation helps you develop a sense of connection to the earth. It is empowering when you are feeling overwhelmed by the "state of the world." It helps environmental activists recharge their batteries and reconnect to the driving force of love.

Allow 10 to 20 minutes.

Find yourself a comfortable sitting position, either seated on the floor or in an upright chair. Sit tall. Feel your connection to the earth beneath you and the sky above you. Tune in to the natural flow of your breath.

Before you begin this meditation, imagine that you are drawing a circle of safety and protection around yourself. You can do this by imagining that you are drawing a circle of light around yourself, silently repeating the phrase, "I surround myself with love and light and I am safe."

Begin by sending loving kindness and good wishes to yourself. Picture yourself happy, healthy, safe, and at ease. Surround yourself with love and compassion.

Now bring to mind a picture of your home, planet Earth. Recall all that you love and find beautiful about the earth: the trees, forests, plants, animals, birds, sea, sky, rivers, and mountains. Cultivate gratitude and love for all that the earth gives you, such as a home, air, food, water, and shelter. Immerse yourself in love and appreciation for the earth's bounty.

As you picture the earth's beauty, be aware of any concerns for her that may arise. If you notice concerns, try to locate where you are feeling them in your body. If any tension is building up, then imagine that you are surrounding that part of your body with love and compassion. Have compassion for the earth and for yourself.

Now begin to silently repeat loving kindness (*metta*) phrases for the earth:

> *May the earth be safe.*
> *May the earth be happy.*
> *May the earth be healthy.*
> *May the earth live with ease.*

As you repeat the loving kindness phrases, imagine that you are sending, love, good wishes, and compassion to the earth.

When you are ready, let go of repeating the phrases.

Now see if you can picture a world where the earth is healed and whole again. Imagine that the planet has healed itself. Its ecosystems are healthy and well balanced again. Earth, air, and water are clean and pure. Allow yourself to enjoy this image of a world where human beings live in harmony with the environment. Send out good wishes, loving kindness, and compassion to all the other human beings who share this planet with you. Send out a wish that all of us might care and look after the earth, our home, with wisdom. Repeat the loving kindness phrases for all beings on earth:

*May we all be safe.*
*May we all be happy.*
*May we all be healthy.*
*May we all live with ease.*

When you are ready, let go of repeating the phrases. Once again surround yourself with love and compassion.

Conclude the meditation by noticing your body's connection to the earth so as to ground yourself. Become aware of your surroundings. Be aware of any insights that you might have gained from doing this meditation. Resolve to take these feelings of love, kindness, and compassion, for yourself, for others, and for the earth, back into your everyday life.

## Tree Wisdom in Autumn

With the arrival of autumn, spending time around trees is the perfect way to connect with the changes occurring in nature. When you are out and about, mindfully observe a tree: the leaves changing color, the textures and shapes of fallen leaves, the sound of leaves underfoot. Watch a leaf fall from a tree. Some people think it lucky to catch a falling leaf.

<hr />

EXERCISE

# Trees and Creativity during Autumn

You can use the time that you have spent mindfully around trees as a springboard for your creativity. If you are stuck for ideas, here are a few to get you going:

- Collect objects that have fallen from trees, such as fir cones, conkers, acorns, and so on, and make a centerpiece for your table or place it in view of the space where you do yoga or meditation.

- Collect a variety of fallen leaves of different shapes and sizes. Use these leaves to inspire an act of creativity, such as these:

  - ⊕ Paint the leaves and print with them.

  - ⊕ Draw around the silhouette of the leaves and cut out the shapes (if you don't have drawing paper, then old newspapers or magazines will do).

  - ⊕ Press the leaves between the pages of a book (protect the book by using two sheets of plain paper to prevent the leaf coming into contact with the print). Put the book under a pile of heavy books, and look again in a few weeks at your dried, pressed leaf (you can do the same with flowers).

- The science behind why leaves fall from the trees in autumn is fascinating. How much do you know about this phenomenon? Use the resources available to you online, in books, from a knowledgeable friend, and so on to find out more. Once you have done this, observe whether your newfound knowledge adds or detracts from your enjoyment and appreciation of trees. Share your knowledge with friends.

- Over the next four weeks, take at least one photo each week of a tree from the same angle. Once you have all your photos, compare them and notice the changes that have occurred in the tree over the four-week period. (Choose a deciduous tree—i.e., one that loses its leaves in autumn.)

- Try out the Autumn Equinox Yoga Practice in this chapter.

## Meditation upon a Sycamore Tree at Autumn Equinox

In our town center is an ancient churchyard. It is an island surrounded by busy, noisy passing traffic, shops, and shoppers. In the churchyard there is a row of tall sycamore trees; they seem so still, serene, and peaceful in contrast to the relentless activity of the town around them. These sycamore trees have taught me to simply *be* in the midst of all the *doing* and to stay at the center of the circle and let all things take their course. Below is the tree prose poem that I wrote in response to meditatively spending time around these trees.

*Around the sycamore tree the city draws a circle of activity. A leaf falls from the tree, down to the river, and on to the sea. The sycamore stays at the center of the circle and lets all things take their course. Life goes on around you; life goes on within you; you and life are one.*

## Autumn Equinox Meditation Questions

These questions are designed to be used around the time of the autumn equinox. It's fine to use them a week or two before or after the actual date of the equinox. Guidance on how to use the seasonal meditation questions can be found in chapter 1.

- Autumn is a time of fruitfulness and harvest.
    - Looking back over the past year, what have I achieved and what is my own personal harvest?
    - What am I harvesting in my personal relationships?
    - Which projects were fruitful and how will I celebrate and build on my success?
    - Which projects failed to bear fruit and how would I do things differently next time to ensure success?
    - How do I thank those people who have helped me realize my harvest?
    - How will I share my harvest with others?
    - How do I cultivate gratitude for all the blessings in my life?

- At the autumn equinox day and night are equal. It also corresponds with the date that the sun enters the sign of Libra, the scales of balance.
    - How does it feel when my life is out of balance? What are the signs to look for?

    ↬ How does it feel when my life is in balance? What's different?

    ↬ In what ways does yoga help me bring balance into my life? Which aspects of yoga have I found helpful for this?

    ↬ Apart from yoga, what do I find helps create balance in my life?

- After the autumn equinox the days will continue to shorten, and we will enter the darkest phase of the year. Now we move from a focus on outward action to one of contemplation and incubation.

    ↬ What do I wish to incubate over the autumn-to-winter season, ready to send up new green shoots next spring?

    ↬ What are the ways in which my yoga practice can nourish, enrich, and support me over the autumn-to-winter months?

    ↬ How will I go about bringing light in to the dark days of winter?

- In preparation for winter the trees are letting go of their leaves.

    ↬ What do I wish to let go of at this time?

    ↬ Are there any habits, ways of being, relationships, and activities, and so on that no longer serve me well? What are the steps I need to take to loosen their hold over me?

    ↬ What's important to me? What do I need to let go of in order to prioritize the things that I value most in life?

    ↬ In what way would letting go of physical clutter improve the quality of life for me and those closest to me?

- In nature nothing is wasted. The leaves that fall from the trees are composted and provide nourishment for the tree over winter. How can I help the earth by wasting less and reusing and recycling more?

    ↬ This autumn how will I connect with nature and take time to appreciate the beauty of the season?

CHAPTER SEVEN

# Autumn Turns to Winter

*End of October to mid-December in the Northern Hemisphere*
*End of April to mid-June in the Southern Hemisphere*

Over the next few weeks the dark will be expanding. The waning cycle of the sun will reach its fullness at the winter solstice, at which point it will end and we will welcome back the return of the light. Our yoga practice offers us many ways of lifting our spirits and lightening up the dark days of autumn and winter.

## Every Ending Is a New Beginning

Autumn is turning to winter now and the leaves are falling from the trees; the days are getting shorter and cold frosty mornings whisper that winter is on the way.

In many traditions the point when we enter the darkest phase of the year is seen as a new beginning rather than an ending. We pass through the darkness only to be reborn into the light at the winter solstice. You and I, before being born into the light of the world, began our lives in the darkness of our mother's womb. An oak tree started out as an acorn buried in the darkness of the soil. Each new day begins and ends in darkness at sunrise and sunset. Every month, before the new moon is reborn into the night sky, there is a period of darkness when the moon is not yet visible. Similarly, as autumn turns to winter, we are entering the darkest phase of the year, until the sun is reborn at the winter solstice in December. Every ending is a new beginning.

In the same way that the darkness of the night gives us rest and dream time, so too the dark half of the year gives us an opportunity to pause, rest, and rejuvenate. Just as the oak tree stays alive over winter by stripping itself of leaves and using almost no energy, we too can look for opportunities during this autumn-to-winter period to enter a place of stillness and simply be utterly present in the moment.

Although this period is not a good time for action, it is the perfect time to plan and incubate ideas; then, like a bulb resting in the soil over winter, you will be ready next spring to send up new green shoots. Spend some time now picturing what you want to get out into the world next growing season and you will be ready to surf the crest of the wave of the growing tide when spring comes round again.

At this time we have Halloween, with its candlelit pumpkin lanterns and children dressed up in spooky outfits trick-or-treating door to door. Traditionally, it's a time for honoring the dead. This can be done through a simple ritual, such as lighting a candle for a meaningful person in your life who has passed on. This might be an ancestor, such as a dearly loved grandparent, or it could be someone who has inspired you and whom you feel a spiritual connection to, such as a writer, poet, painter, singer, political agitator, or yogini. In yoga the root chakra (*muladhara*) is associated with ancestral connections and a sense of tribal belonging.

How we are remembered by our descendants will depend on how we act today. Our kindnesses and cruelties echo down the generations. We don't want to hand on a poison chalice of meanness and petty grudges; rather, let us hand down a torch of love. What do you consider your heirloom gifts to be? And what do you wish to pass on to the next generation?

Although it's natural to be afraid of the dark, our spiritual practice trains us to turn and face our fear in order that its hold over us might be diminished. Our yoga and mindfulness practice can help us embrace and engage with our fears, moving through them and out into the light again.

## Welcoming the Composting Phase of the Year

If the period between late autumn and the winter solstice were a phase of the moon, it would be the Balsamic Moon, which is the waning crescent moon. The predominant quality (*guna*) of the autumn-to-winter season is that of heaviness, darkness, dormancy, and decay (*tamas*). And whereas it is easy to love the beauty of the red, yellow, orange, and crimson autumn leaves, it is harder to enthuse over piles of sodden old brown leaves that are dying back. Although the composting phase of the year is not pretty, it is an essential part of the circle of life.

The Buddha reminds us that a lotus cannot flower if its roots are resting upon marble. In order to flower the lotus needs to be rooted in mud. There is a partnership between the beauty of the lotus flower and the mud; they go together hand in hand. Likewise, the old brown leaves rotting down in winter provide the compost that gives us new green leaves and blossom in spring.

Traditionally, the autumn-to-winter phase of the year is associated with old age. As we confront the death of the year, we also come face to face with our own mortality, and although this can be uncomfortable, it also presents us with the opportunity for spiritual growth.

The Buddha encouraged his monks and nuns to go to the charnel ground to receive a lesson in impermanence by contemplating the body of someone who had recently died. It's unlikely that we would go to such extremes in our own meditation practice. However, our seasonal practice offers us a gentler way of working with the cycle of life, death, and rebirth by observing the annual cycle of composting, decay, and rebirth. We too are part of nature and we can observe our own reactions to the natural process of aging, in ourselves and others, and the patterns of clinging or avoidance that this brings up in us.

When I started yoga in as a teenager in the 1970s, yoga books made wild claims that yoga would give you eternal youth and even immortality! In the Yoga Sutras Patanjali states that supernatural powers (*siddhi*), which include bodily perfection, eternal youth, and immortality, can be acquired through the practice of yogic discipline. He also gives a warning that we should not become too mesmerized by these powers, or they will become a distraction from the ultimate aim of yoga, which is enlightenment (Yoga Sutra 3.37).

Whereas it's true that yoga can help us maintain our youthful vigor, it becomes an unhealthy pursuit when it morphs into clinging to something that all of us must ultimately surrender. From this point of view, it's understandable why in the Yoga Sutras Patanjali identifies the will to live (*abhinivesa*) as one of the obstacles preventing the yogi from reaching enlightenment (Yoga Sutra 2.9). Although the survival instinct is entirely natural and desirable, it becomes pernicious when it develops into a denial of reality and an obsession with preserving youth at any cost. By reconnecting us to the simplicity and beauty of the eternal cycle of life, death, and renewal, our seasonal awareness helps us grow into spiritual maturity.

There is a multibillion-dollar industry built around preserving youthful vitality and freezing it in time. The media loves that which is young and beautiful, whereas that which is old, unattractive, and "past its prime" is edited out and absent from our screens, newspapers, and magazines. Women especially are told that it is wrong for them to blossom into the splendor of their full maturity; they must stay preserved in aspic in the spring and summer of their days. Fortunately, Nature is not so squeamish about aging, as it is an essential part of her design for a thriving, healthy ecosystem.

Scientists studying forests are only just now beginning to understand the important contribution dead wood makes to the health of the forest. Standing dead trees and fallen debris provide a fantastic array of "microhabitats" for woodland wildlife. A dead tree is said to support more diversity of life than a living one, including homes for birds, bats, invertebrates, plants, and fungi.[21] Eventually the tree decomposes into humus that nourishes growing young trees and replenishes the forest.

We humans are learning to tolerate the "untidiness" of fallen and decaying wood and resist the urge to clear it away, which in the long term is detrimental to the health of the forest. Now that we understand the importance of dead wood in our forests, can we make a leap of understanding and recognize the importance of "dead wood" in our own personal life? We tend to like our lives to be ordered and tidy. Often, we turn to activities such as yoga to "purify" our lives of all the chaos. We especially do not like the messiness and wildness of raw emotion. And yet perhaps we do need these wild "dead wood" aspects of our lives to maintain the health and well-being of our own personal ecosystem.

The wheel of the year is a mandala and within this circle are to be found sunshine and shadow, light and dark, calm and storm, new life and decay. Our lives too are mandalas and within the circle of our life are to be found sunshine and shadow; highs and lows; happiness and sadness; gains and losses; birth and death. As we develop and hone our seasonal awareness, we learn to be open and present to the wisdom that is contained within every aspect of each season. The buds unfurling on the tree in spring and the

---

21. Peter Wohlleben, *The Hidden Life of Trees: What They Feel, How They Communicate; Discoveries from a Secret World* (Vancouver, BC, Canada: Greystone Books, 2015), 132–35.

old brown leaves in autumn are all part of the same circle. Likewise, a mature spiritual practice enables us to welcome the totality of every aspect of our life as part of the circle.

## We Light a Candle in the Darkness

Our challenge during the autumn-winter period is on the one hand to embrace the darkness and on the other to bring light into the darkness. We recognize how darkness offers us rest, regeneration, and renewal during the autumn-winter months. At the same time, it's important to lighten up dark days by conjuring up healing images of light.

In Classical Yoga the divine spark within is called the *Atman*, and it is said to be like a flame or a continuously burning pilot light that has been ignited in the heart-space. As Nature (*prakriti*) enters her decaying, composting phase, we can counterbalance the dark, heavy (*tamas*) quality of the season by visualizing sattvic images of light and luminescence. We light a candle in the darkness, drawing our awareness inward to contemplate that which is eternal and unchanging.

We can also draw inspiration from Diwali, the Hindu festival of lights, which takes place in late October to early November. *Diwali* means "a row of lights" and marks new beginnings. The Hindu goddess Lakshmi only visits houses that are clean and well lit, so at Diwali Hindu houses are lit with dozens of flickering, hand-painted terracotta lamps.

The Autumn to Winter Yoga Practice that follows shows you how you can bring warmth and creativity into your yoga this autumn-to-winter by inviting the sun to power your practice. Introducing images of the sun into a yoga session can be uplifting and empowering and can expand your sense of what's possible. At the start of your yoga practice, spend some time either lying or sitting and visualize where you can locate or sense the sun in your body. The solar plexus, at the center of the body, is a particularly good area to choose for this visualization. Then, as you do your yoga practice, keep bringing your awareness back to this part of the body and visualize a sun radiating warmth and light there.

The Spring-Flowering Bulb Meditation later in this chapter uses the image of a bulb resting in the darkness of the soil. Like the bulb, we too can use this period to put down strong roots, find rest and renewal, and incubate ideas, sending up green shoots and blooming next spring.

You might also want to mindfully plant a few spring bulbs, either outside in the soil or inside in a pot. As you place the bulbs in the soil, imagine that you are planting seeds of hope and intention for yourself and your loved ones. Then, as autumn turns to winter, you can enjoy the magic of green shoots appearing through the soil, buds appearing, and flowers blooming.

The autumn-to-winter period is the perfect time to draw inward and reconnect with your inner light. In this way we uncover an illuminating presence that will sustain us through the highs and lows of a life constantly in flux. This is a lamplight that burns steady, in a place where no wind blows.

## Autumn to Winter Yoga Practice

The main theme of this practice is one of bringing light into the darkness and brightening up the dark days of autumn and winter. Sun imagery is used to lift the mood and shake off seasonal blues.

The practice honors the autumn-to-winter urge to hibernate by including poses that draw the awareness inward, such as Standing Twist, forward bends, and Child's Pose.

To avoid the autumn-to-winter slump we include backbends to open the chest. As a nod to Halloween we choose the scary Lion Pose, which is reminiscent of a church gargoyle that scares away evil spirits.

This practice is designed to be used during late autumn to early winter, but it's fine to use it any time of year. The practice has a calming, soothing effect. It is gently energizing and boosts the mood, encouraging a sunny outlook.

Allow 20 to 30 minutes.

### 1. Standing Like a Tree
Stand tall, feet parallel and about hip width apart. Be aware of the contact between your feet and the earth beneath you. Imagine a string attached to the crown of your head, gently pulling you skyward, and simultaneously feel your heels rooting down into the earth. Imagine that you have roots from the soles of your feet going deep down into the earth. Each time you inhale imagine that you are drawing up vital energy (*prana*) from the earth. Picture this energy traveling, like an electric current, up your legs to your power center at the belly (*hara*). Each time you exhale imagine that you are storing this energy at your *hara*. Repeat for 3 to 6 breaths.

Now picture the sun in the sky and then picture a warm, glowing sun at your solar plexus, radiating warmth and light.

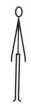

Standing Like a Tree

## 2. Lion Pose (*Simhasana*) standing

Move your legs wider than shoulder width, toes turned slightly out. Bend your arms and make tight fists with your hands. Screw up your face, eyes shut tight. As you exhale, bend the knees, lean forward slightly, and open your mouth wide as you stretch out your tongue, making a *ha* sound as you expel the breath. At the same time, open your eyes wide and spread your fingers wide. As you inhale, straighten the legs and come back to the starting position with clenched fists. Repeat 4 times.

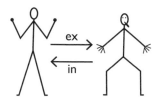

Lion Pose standing

## 3. Standing Twist (*Parivrtti Trikonasana*) Combination sequence

Move the legs wide apart, feet parallel, with the arms out to the side and parallel to the floor. Exhale and come into a Standing Twist (*Parivrtti Trikonasana*) by bending forward from the hip joints, taking one hand to the floor (or to the leg for gentler pose) and raising the other arm up toward the ceiling; look up at the raised hand. Stay here for one breath, lengthening through the spine as you twist. Inhale and come back up to standing, arms out to sides. Repeat on the other side. Inhale and come back up to standing, arms out to sides. Exhale and bend forward from the hip joint, into Wide-Leg Standing

Forward Bend Pose (*Prasarita Padottanasana*), bringing the hands to the floor (for a gentler version, bring the hands to rest on the legs). Inhale and come back up to standing, arms out to sides. Repeat the entire Standing Twist Combination sequence 3 more times.

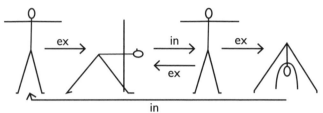

Standing Twist Combination

### 4. Cat Pose to Child's Pose (*Balasana*) with humming

Come onto all fours. On the exhale, hum the breath out, rounding the back up and sitting back into Child's Pose. Inhale and come back to all fours. Repeat 8 times.

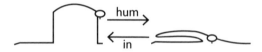

Cat Pose to Child's Pose with humming

### 5. Half-Locust Pose (*Ardha Salabhasana*)

Lie on your front, arms by your sides. Inhale to prepare. As you exhale, lift the head and chest from the floor, sweeping the arms out to the sides like a bird's wings and lifting one straight leg a little way from the floor (keep both frontal hip bones on the floor and do not twist the pelvis). Inhale and lift the chest a little higher. Exhale and lower yourself back to the floor. Repeat on the other side. Repeat 4 times each side.

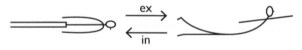

Half-Locust Pose

### 6. Sphinx Pose (*Salamba Bhujangasana*)

Lying on your front, come up into a gentle backbend, propping yourself up on your forearms. Remember not to crease the back of the neck. Feel the tailbone and the crown of the head lengthening away from each other. Be aware of the natural rhythm of the breath. Imagine that there is candle flame at the breastbone radiating out light and warmth. Stay here for a few breaths.

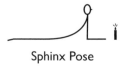

Sphinx Pose

### 7. Child's Pose (*Balasana*)

Rest here for a few breaths.

Child's Pose

### 8. Seated Sun Visualization

Find a comfortable sitting position. Picture a warm, glowing sun at your solar plexus radiating warmth and light. On each exhale, silently chant *Ram* (pronounced *rum*). Repeat 6 times. (*Ram* is the seed mantra associated with the solar plexus chakra, *manipura*. This is a fiery chakra associated with personal power and self-confidence.)

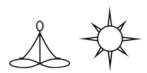

Seated Sun Visualization

### 9. Seated Forward Bend (*Paschimottanasana*) with chanting

Sit tall, legs outstretched (bend the knees to ease the pose) and arms raised. Picture a warm, glowing sun at your solar plexus, radiating warmth and light. Inhale, and as you exhale, fold forward over the legs, chanting *Ram*. Inhale and return to starting position. Repeat 6 times. Then stay in the forward bend for a few breaths, silently chanting.

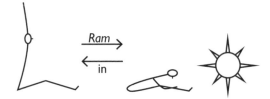

Seated Forward Bend with chanting

## 10. Bridge Pose (*Setu Bandhasana*) with arm movements

Lie on your back, both knees bent, both feet on the floor hip width apart, hands resting on solar plexus. Picture a warm, glowing sun at your solar plexus, radiating warmth and light. Inhale and peel the back from the floor up into Bridge Pose (*Setu Bandhasana*), simultaneously taking the arms out to the sides and onto the floor, just below shoulder level, palms facing up. Stay one breath. Exhale and return to the starting position. Repeat 6 times.

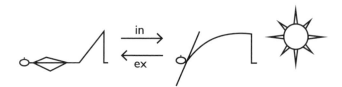

Bridge Pose with arm movements

## 11. Knees-to-Chest Pose (*Apanasana*)

Rest for a few breaths with the knees on the chest.

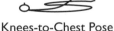

Knees-to-Chest Pose

## 12. Spring-Flowering Bulb Visualization

See page 125. If you prefer, choose another relaxation or meditation.

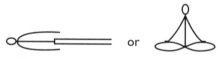

Spring-Flowering Bulb Visualization

## Autumn to Winter Yoga Practice Overview

1. Standing Like a Tree. Inhale: draw up energy from the earth. Exhale: store that energy at your belly (*hara*). Repeat for 3–6 breaths. Picture the sun in the sky and then a warm, glowing sun at your solar plexus.

2. Lion Pose. Make a *ha* sound as you stretch your tongue out. Repeat × 4.

3. Standing Twist Combination sequence. Repeat × 4.

4. Cat Pose to Child's Pose. Exhale: hum breath out, rounding the back up and sitting back into Child's Pose. Inhale: come back to all fours. Repeat × 8.

5. Half-Locust Pose. Repeat × 4 on each side.

6. Sphinx Pose. Imagine candle flame at breastbone radiating light and warmth. Stay for a few breaths.

7. Child's Pose. Rest for a few breaths.

8. Seated Sun Visualization. Picture a warm, glowing sun at solar plexus radiating warmth and light. Exhale: silently chant *Ram*. Repeat × 6.

9. Seated Forward Bend with chanting. Picture a warm, glowing sun at solar plexus. Exhale: fold forward, chanting *Ram*. Inhale: return to starting position. Repeat × 6. Then stay in forward bend for a few breaths, silently chanting.

10. Bridge Pose with arm movements. Picture a warm, glowing sun at solar plexus. Inhale: come up into Bridge Pose. Stay one breath. Exhale: return to starting position. Repeat × 6.

11. Knees-to-Chest Pose. Rest for a few breaths.

12. Spring-Flowering Bulb Visualization.

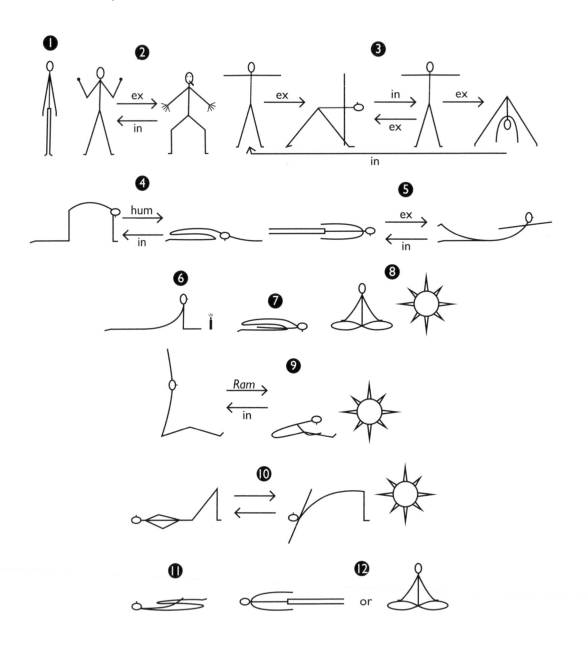

## EXERCISE
# Spring-Flowering Bulb Visualization

This visualization reminds us that although nature lies dormant over winter, under the surface there is still a lot happening. The visualization will lighten up the autumn-winter days and give us hope for the renewal that comes with the arrival of spring. It is also a metaphor for the work over autumn and winter that we ourselves do to incubate hopes and dreams for the future.

Allow about 10 minutes.

Find yourself a comfortable position, either sitting or lying. Relax your shoulders down away from your ears and soften your face with a half smile. Become aware of the natural flow of your breath.

Imagine that you are in a beautiful garden in autumn. It's a place where you feel safe and peaceful. Look around—what do you see? Notice the colors, shapes, textures, and fragrances of the autumnal garden.

Imagine that you have come to the garden to plant spring-flowering bulbs. Picture yourself picking up a bulb and holding it in your hand. Notice its shape, color, and texture. Picture yourself picking up your trowel and digging a hole in the soil. Notice the color and feel of the soil. Now picture placing the bulb in the soil and covering it with soil. And then you water the soil around where it is planted.

There is a chill in the air and the wind is blowing leaves around the garden. Even though you can sense winter is on its way, your heart is warmed when you think of your bulb snug in the soil. Soon it will put down roots and then will lie dormant in the darkness of the soil over the cold months ahead. In time, when the weather starts to warm up again, the bulb will draw on its store of energy and send up leaves and a stem, and eventually it will flower. Picture in your mind's eye the beauty of your flower in bloom in spring, shimmering in a gentle breeze.

When you are ready, let go of the image of the flower and garden. Become aware of your body again and notice where it is in contact with the floor or your support and the sensations associated with this.

Now take a few minutes to consider what you will be incubating in your life over the coming months, ready to send up green shoots next spring.

Bring your awareness back to your surroundings. Resolve to take any positive insights that you have gained from this visualization back into your everyday life. Then when you are ready, carry on with your day.

## The Surrounding a Difficulty with Love Meditation

In this chapter we have considered how the autumn-to-winter period gives us the opportunity, as we enter the darkest phase of the year, to turn and face our fears. The Surrounding a Difficulty with Love Meditation will help you develop the skills to tolerate and embrace difficult emotions more easily. This in turn will help you build up courage and emotional resilience.

In this meditation we learn to approach our difficulties with curiosity rather than avoid them, and this can help reduce the intensity and duration of difficult emotions. This meditation can also help you to learn how to show love and acceptance to yourself when you are suffering.

If you are new to meditation, before you try this one, it would be best to gain experience with some of the less challenging exercises in this book, such as Calming Cloud Meditation (chapter 2), the Loving Kindness Walking Meditation (chapter 3), Placing Thoughts on a Leaf Visualisation (chapter 6), or the Four-Minute Check-In Meditation (chapter 8). If you are suffering from clinical depression or severe anxiety, wait until you are feeling well again before trying it.

Allow 10 to 20 minutes.

Find yourself a comfortable sitting position, either on the floor or in a straight-backed chair. Have a tall, erect, and relaxed posture. Or if you prefer, this meditation can be done lying down.

Notice where your body is in contact with the floor or your support. Allow those parts of your body that are in contact with the floor or your support to go with gravity and relax down into the earth.

Take your awareness around your body, noticing which parts of your body already feel relaxed and which parts feel tight or tense. Let go of any unnecessary tension, relax your shoulders down away from your ears, and soften your face with a half smile. Become aware of the natural flow of your breath.

Now bring to mind a difficulty that has been troubling you. Don't choose the most difficult problem in your life; rather, start off by focusing on a minor worry or concern. Spend a few minutes turning this troubling situation over in your mind. Notice in a non-judgmental way any thoughts and feelings that are arising in response to this difficulty.

As you dwell on this troubling situation, notice how your body is responding. Notice where you are feeling the difficulty most strongly in your body. Rather than pushing the unpleasant sensations away, see if you can welcome and surround them with love. Imagine that you are giving a big hug to the parts of your body that have tightened or tensed up in response to this troubling emotion.

Notice how the intense physical sensations change from moment to moment. Keep surrounding them with love. As you breathe in, imagine that you are breathing into this part of your body. As you exhale, soften and release, letting go of any tightness or tension.

Now let go of focusing on this difficult situation and the emotions it brings up for you. Bring your awareness back to where your body is in contact with the floor or your support. Feel yourself supported by the earth.

Become aware of sounds inside the room and sounds outside. Come back to an awareness of your surroundings. Notice how you are feeling now and in what way this is different from how you felt at the start of the meditation. Give yourself a big hug and then carry on with your day.

## Tree Wisdom in Autumn to Winter

As autumn turns to winter, the prettiness of autumn leaves changes to the brown, soggy mess of decomposing leaves. Mindfulness encourages us to turn toward and embrace all aspects of our experience non-judgmentally. When you are out and about during this season, take time to notice how trees manifest both the beauty of the season and the process of decomposition that is occurring. Mindfully observe what feelings arise in you in response to both the beautiful and the decaying. Is it possible to find richness in both aspects of the season? Approach this mindfulness exercise with an open mind and curiosity. Use all your senses to appreciate the season in its fullness.

EXERCISE

# Trees and Creativity
## during Autumn to Winter

You can use the time that you have spent mindfully around trees as a springboard for your creativity. If you are stuck for ideas, here are a few to start you off:

- Take a series of photos contrasting the beauty of the season and its composting aspect. For example, you might take a photo of some beautiful red yew berries and another photo of windfall apples bruised and decomposing on the ground.

- Write about five things you like about this time of year and five things you dislike.

- How much do you know about the vital importance of old, decaying trees in the ecosystem? Use the resources available to you online, in books, from a knowledgeable friend, and so on to find out more. Once you have done this, observe whether your newfound knowledge adds to or detracts from your enjoyment and appreciation of trees. Share your knowledge with friends.

- Too much tidiness in a garden is bad for wildlife. Designate part of your garden (if you have one) as a less tidy, wildlife-friendly area.

## Meditation upon a Yew Tree

Whenever possible I prefer to walk and leave the car at home. One of my well-trodden routes takes me through a churchyard where an ancient yew tree grows. The tree's branches curve down to the ground and then grow back up again in a U-bend, which creates a house-like space around the bough of the tree. Yew trees are often found in churchyards, and it is believed that the trees marked sacred sites where people gathered to worship before the churches were even built.[22] In the name of research for this book, I persuaded my husband to take a midnight walk with me to visit my favorite yew tree under the light of the full moon. It was that starry, moonlit walk through the churchyard that inspired the tree prose poem below.

---

22. Barbara G. Walker, *The Woman's Dictionary of Symbols and Sacred Objects* (New York: HarperCollins Publishers, 1988), 476.

*I am the tree of the full moon. Stars dance above and below me. I am the church of the night sky. My tree children form a constellation around me, our heads bowed together in holy communion, making sacred vows of love. As above so below; my roots, an earthly mirror of my heavenly branches, find succor in Mother Earth.*

*I am the evergreen Tree of Eternity:* Taxus baccata, *the yew tree. I am the Tree of the Dark Moon, before the crescent moon has appeared in the night sky. I am the dark night before hope arises with the new dawn.*

*My leaves are eaten by the satin beauty moth. My seeds, leaves, and bark are all extremely poisonous. Turn toward that which you most fear. In skillful hands poison becomes the medicine that cures whatever ails you. Walk toward the darkness and come through to the light.*

*My branches are kindly old hands cupping all your cares and woes. They are a loving arm wrapped around your life. Together we can transform fear into love. Here, take this courage and step inside the mandala of your life and be renewed.*

*Over the years, tears have been shed and flowers placed on newly carved headstones. I am the Tree of the Mourning Moon. The lesson of the Mourning Moon is that we mourn, but then mourning comes to an end: a new start, a fresh start. Your roots are my roots; my renewal is your renewal. I am the tree of Life-in-Death: endings and new beginnings. When you go, what is left behind? All that is left is love: so be kind.*

*I am the Tree of Resurrection. Blackbirds eat my fleshy red arils and disperse the black seeds there within. In spring snowdrops carpet the floor of my womb-like treehouse. In summer white-flowered brambles weave around my branches, which bow down and take root in the earth, and I am renewed.*

## Autumn to Winter Meditation Questions

These questions are designed to be used any time from around the end of October to mid-November in the Northern Hemisphere and from around the end of April to mid-May in the Southern Hemisphere. Guidance on how to use the seasonal meditation questions can be found in chapter 1.

- As winter approaches, who brings warmth and light into my life?
  - ↬ How will I express my gratitude to them?
  - ↬ As the leaves fall from the trees, what do I need to let go of in order to have the time and energy to nurture these key relationships?
  - ↬ How can I bring warmth, light, and joy into the lives of my loved ones over the coming winter?

- Looking back over the past year, what have I achieved (in work, home, study, etc.)?

- Although the autumn-to-winter period is not a good time for action, it's a great time for planning. What plans do I have for next year? (Work, home, holidays, relationships, adventures, etc.)
  - ↬ What do I wish to incubate over the winter, ready to send up fresh, new green shoots in the spring?
  - ↬ Which projects do I wish to nurture and nourish, ready to launch into the world next spring, and so take full advantage of the growing season energy?
  - ↬ If I were to imagine a world where anything is possible, what would I envisage my future to be?

- To conserve energy during the winter months trees are letting go of their leaves.
  - ↬ What do I wish to let go of?
  - ↬ What needs processing and composting?

- The autumn-to-winter period is a time of drawing inward, resting, and recuperating.
  - ↬ How will I go about nurturing and nourishing myself over the winter?
  - ↬ Which yoga practices will energize me and help banish the winter blues?

↬ Which activities nourish me and which activities deplete me? How can I increase the nourishing activities and reduce the depleting ones?

• How do I feel about moving into the darkest phase of the year?
   ↬ Am I able to lovingly hold my natural fear of darkness while at the same time recognizing the potential of darkness to offer rest and healing?
   ↬ Am I using up valuable energy resisting and avoiding things that I fear? Are there any small steps that I could take to enable me to turn and face my fears?
   ↬ How can I bring light into the darkness?

• In many traditions this is a time for honoring ancestors. (For our purpose "ancestors" could be blood relatives, or it could be people from the past whom you admire and to whose lineage you feel a spiritual connection.)
   ↬ How can I honor those who have gone before me and thank them for the gifts that they have bequeathed to me?
   ↬ How would I like to be remembered, and what gifts do I want to hand down to future generations?
   ↬ Are there any older members of my family (or lineage) whom I could talk to and find out more about our family history?

• In order to cope better with the winter months ahead, what can I learn from nature about adaptability and versatility?
   ↬ How can I help and protect wildlife over the winter?
   ↬ How will I go about getting out and enjoying the beauty of the season?

CHAPTER EIGHT

# Winter Solstice

*December 20–23 in the Northern Hemisphere*
*June 20–23 in the Southern Hemisphere*

The winter solstice marks the shortest day of the year. We have arrived at the point in the year when the darkness has expanded to its fullness and must now bow down to the sun. It is a time of hope and a time to dream the life you wish for into being. During the remaining winter months, your yoga practice can help banish the winter blues, boost your mood, and support and energize you.

## Hope Is Reborn at the Winter Solstice

The sun, reborn at the winter solstice, is like a new moon: the first few days of the moon's waxing cycle the new moon is not yet visible in the sky; in the same way, at the winter solstice, it is not immediately evident that the light has returned. Winter stretches out before us, the sun is low in the sky and casts long shadows, and summer still seems a far-off dream. However, although it is not apparent to us yet, the earth's energy has shifted from darkness to light, moon to sun, yin to yang, water to fire, inner to outer, and from contemplation to action.

In Latin *sol* means "sun" and *sistere* means "to stand still." Here at the winter solstice the sun appears to stand still before it changes direction. We too stand still; we pause and look back over the journey that we have taken over the dark half of the year. This has been a journey that follows a path spiraling inward to the center of our being. And now we reflect upon what we have learned along the way and consider what wisdom we will be taking with us into the new solar year. Like the sun we stand still and prepare to change direction. We turn our face to the sun and look toward the path that spirals back out into the world.

Over the past few months we have been incubating ideas; now the time is approaching to take action and get our ideas out into the world, a time for pushing rather than for yielding. Whatever seeds you plant during the growing season will, like the returning light, expand and grow. So, it pays to know what you want to *do* in the months ahead, and then you will be well placed to ride the crest of the wave of growing season energy. Before you step into the new year, take the time to consider what you wish to bring out into the light over the coming year.

Sometimes, with no effort on our part, a dream comes true. However, most of the time we need to take action to make the fairy-tale ending become a reality. At the winter solstice we pause to consider what we need to do to make our dreams come true. We plan what actions we will be taking during the fertile half of the year.

Now is a good time to consider what your hopes and dreams are for the year ahead. If you have become estranged from your dreams, take some time to get to know them again. As the sun returns at the winter solstice, this is the perfect time to ask, what lights my fire? Make a list of all the things you love doing and that bring you pleasure. This might seem a bit scary if you are out of the habit of taking time for yourself. Start small, choose something from your list that's easy to do, and do it! This will build your confidence, and you will be able to build on your successes. Reignite those hidden passions and dare to dream the life you want to live.

## We Welcome Back the Sun and Prepare for Action

The new solar year has begun; the light is expanding, and the days will gradually lengthen again. The light will continue to expand up until the summer solstice in June, when, having reached its fullness, it will once again begin to wane. The time for action is approaching, but it is not here yet.

On a spiritual level we create a sacred space at the solstice by pausing and taking time to reflect on, and connect with, the light within, enabling us to radiate warmth and sunshine out into the dark days of winter. Following the solstice, as you spiral back out into the world, let your actions be guided by this divine lamplight. Bring your awareness back to it whenever you feel alone, troubled, confused, or are at a crossroads and uncertain about which path to take. In the coming growing season, resolve to stay connected to this inner light and then everything you do will be illuminated and guided by your inner wisdom. What do you want to bring out into the light over the coming months?

Our challenge over the coming season will be to stay connected to our inner wisdom while taking action out in the world. One way to invest your actions with meaning is to be clear in your heart what your values are. What really matters to you? What do you care about? What are your guiding principles? Who's important to you and how will you show them you care? Our values are like the sun: if we place them at the center of our life, then our actions can revolve around them. When our values are the axis around which our actions rotate, then our lives are inspired with warmth, light, beauty, and meaning.

It is helpful to differentiate between goals and values. Goals are focused on an endpoint, whereas values are more about the process. Goals can be very helpful when you want to get from A to B. However, if we get too goal-orientated, we may forget to enjoy the journey. Values are more about a direction of travel. They allow us to do the work and to let go of the outcome. Our values inform the way that we respond to whatever arises in our life and how we treat ourselves and those around us.

We live a life of freedom when we live a life inspired by our values. The final chapter of Patanjali's Yoga Sutras looks at the subject of absolute freedom (*kaivalya*). The discipline of the yogic path leads ultimately to this goal of spiritual liberation.

The pause at the solstice is a good time to contemplate on the nature of freedom. Has your practice of yoga, or another spiritual discipline, given you a taste, or a glimpse, of what absolute freedom (*kaivalya*) might be like? If so, how would you describe this state of liberation? If you have not directly experienced it, can you imagine what it might be like, and is it something that you would aspire to?

Sometimes the relentless pace of our lives can leave us feeling trapped within a wheel of perpetual activity. At the winter solstice we take the time to pause and reflect before we step over the threshold and into the new year. And within this pause lies freedom.

## Winter Solstice Yoga to Awaken the Light Within

The newly conceived light at the solstice is a seed born into darkness. During the autumn and winter, nature's most predominant quality is that of *tamas*, the black strand of creation, embodying darkness and heaviness. The positive side of *tamas* energy is that it has a grounding effect and it makes us rest and recuperate after the frenetic activity of the growing season. The negative side of *tamas* is that it can make us feel heavy, lethargic, and prone to the winter blues.

If you are someone who makes New Year's resolutions and finds it hard to take the action to follow them through, it's probably due to the lingering predominance of winter's *tamas* energy. Once you can recognize the pattern of this energy at play in yourself and your environment, you'll be able to work more effectively with it. You can make allowance for the fact that due to the prevalence of *tamas*, it takes all of us a while to shake off hibernation mode and get our year into gear.

Your yoga practice can help you to counteract the tamasic lethargy and depression associated with the season by bringing light in to the darkness. Also, you can honor the natural tendency to want to stay in hibernation by choosing restful, restorative (*langhana*) yoga poses such as Child's Pose (*Balasana*), Knees-to-Chest Pose (*Apanasana*), Seated Forward Bend (*Paschimottanasana*), and Tortoise Pose (*Kurmasana*).

You can lift your spirits, boost your happy hormones, and ward off winter blues by choosing energizing (*brahmana*) techniques including lengthening the inhale and the pause following the inhale. You can avoid the winter slump by including energizing, uplifting, expansive poses such as Cobra Pose (*Bhujangasana*), Locust Pose (*Salabhasana*), Warrior Poses (*Virabhadrasana*), Bow Pose (*Dhanurasana*), Camel Pose (*Ustrasana*), the Dancer Pose (*Natarajasana*), Bridge Pose (*Setu Bandhasana*), Upward-Facing Dog Pose (*Urdhva Muka Svanasana*), and Sphinx Pose (*Salamba Bhujangasana*).

As the days start to get longer and lighter, the dark, heavy quality of *tamas* will begin to subside. The quality of *rajas* then becomes more prevalent. *Rajas* is the red thread of creation that supports activity, action, and creativity. You can use your busy, restless *rajas* energy to spur you on to take some small steps toward achieving the goals that you laid out in your New Year's resolutions. Also, *rajas* loves planning, so now is a great time to make a list of all the things you want to do and achieve this year.

The rebirth of the light at the winter solstice is a sattvic moment. *Sattva* is the white thread of creation, and it is the quality associated with lucidity, clarity, purity, and light.[23] At the solstice the light is just like a pinprick of light streaming into a darkened room, but over the coming weeks and months the light will expand until the room is flooded with shafts of bright sunlight. Whether you are old or young, you will sense that sattvic shift of energy that occurs at the solstice and you will feel a sense of hope stirring deep within you with the return of the sun.

Before long the first spring flowers, white, yellow, and golden, will appear, bringing light into the darkness and heralding that spring is on the way. Over the coming growing season our challenge will be to stay connected to this light, clear sattvic energy within, so that all our actions are guided by our inner wisdom. At the winter solstice we pause to celebrate the pure sattvic quality of the light reborn, and we create a space within our heart to welcome back the newborn light.

## Winter Solstice Yoga Practice: Winter Solstice Salute to the Sun

Performing rounds of Salute to the Sun (*Surya Namaskar*) is a wonderful way to welcome back the sun at the winter solstice. *Surya* means "sun" and *Namaskar* means "to bow to."

The seasons were very important to ancient people, hunter-gatherers, who were out in all weathers, and some even worshipped the sun. The Norse people, in days gone by, saw the sun as a wheel that changed the seasons. Salute to the Sun is also like a wheel in that it is a circular yoga sequence that celebrates the sun.

You can bring warmth into a cold winter's day by picturing a warm glowing sun at your solar plexus as you perform this Salute to the Sun.

This sequence will get your circulation going, which boosts your immune system. It's energizing and helps you shake off winter lethargy. It boosts your mood and banishes the winter blues.

You can perform as many rounds of the Salute to the Sun as you wish. You can also play about with varying the speed of the sequence. It can be very soothing if performed slowly and meditatively. Try staying and resting for a few breaths in Downward-Facing

---

23. Barbara G. Walker, *The Woman's Encyclopedia of Myths and Secrets* (New York: HarperCollins Publishers, 1983), 358.

Dog Pose, Child's Pose, and Standing Forward Bend. In this way your Salute to the Sun becomes like a moving prayer.

### 1. Mountain Pose (*Tadasana*) with Sun Visualization

Stand in Mountain Pose (*Tadasana*), hands in Prayer Position (*Namaste*). In your mind's eye picture the sun rising in the sky. Now picture a warm, glowing sun at your solar plexus, radiating warmth and light, and keep this image in mind as you perform the Salute to the Sun.

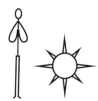

Mountain Pose with Sun Visualization

### 2. Mountain Pose (*Tadasana*) into Standing Forward Bend (*Uttanasana*)

From Mountain Pose raise your arms out to the sides and up above your head, then come down into a Standing Forward Bend (*Uttanasana*).

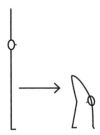

Mountain Pose into Standing Forward Bend

### 3. Bend knees and arch back

Bend the knees and arch the back, and then come back down into the forward bend.

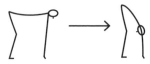

Bend knees and arch back

## 4. Plank Pose (*Chaturanga Dandasana*)

Step the legs back, one at a time, into Plank Pose (*Chaturanga Dandasana*), positioning the whole body in one long line.

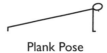

Plank Pose

## 5. Side Plank (*Vasisthasana*)

From Plank Pose swivel to one side into Side Plank (*Vasisthasana*). Repeat on the other side.

*For a gentler practice, skip Side Plank and go straight to step 6.*

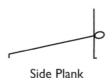

Side Plank

## 6. Plank Pose (*Chaturanga Dandasana*) into Child's Pose (*Balasana*)

Come back into Plank Pose and drop the knees to the floor, sitting back into Child's Pose (*Balasana*). Rest here for a few breaths.

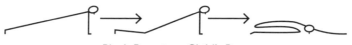

Plank Pose into Child's Pose

## 7. Child's Pose (*Balasana*) into Upward-Facing Dog (*Urdhva Mukha Svanasana*)

From Child's Pose come into Upward-Facing Dog (*Urdhva Mukha Svanasana*).

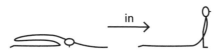

Child's Pose into Upward-Facing Dog

### 8. Downward-Facing Dog (*Adho Mukha Svanasana*)

From Upward-Facing Dog turn the toes under and swing back into a Downward-Facing Dog Pose (*Adho Mukha Svanasana*). Stay for a few breaths in the pose.

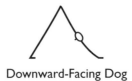

Downward-Facing Dog

### 9. Lunge Pose (*Anjaneyasana*)

From Downward-Facing Dog Pose bring your right foot forward into Lunge Pose (*Anjaneyasana*).

Lunge Pose

### 10. Standing Forward Bend (*Uttanasana*) into arched back

Bring the other foot forward, coming into a Standing Forward Bend. Bend the knees and arch the back.

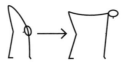

Standing Forward Bend into arched back

### 11. Standing Forward Bend (*Uttanasana*) into standing

Come back into the Forward Bend and stay for a few breaths. Then sweep the arms out to the sides and up above the head, coming back up to standing.

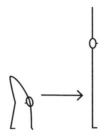

Standing Forward Bend into standing

## 12. Mountain Pose (*Tadasana*) with Sun Visualization

Bring the hands back into the Prayer Position (*Namaste*) and rest here for a few breaths. As you rest, picture in your mind's eye the sun rising in the sky. And then picture a warm, glowing sun at your solar plexus, radiating warmth and light, and keep this image in mind as you perform another round of the Salute to the Sun. Take this warm, sunny glow into your next activity and into the rest of your day!

Mountain Pose with Sun Visualization

For a gentler practice, instead of Salute to the Sun, do a few rounds of Albatross Sequence 2 (see the Winter to Spring Yoga Practice in the next chapter). This Albatross Sequence 2 can also be used as a warm-up for Salute to the Sun.

For a longer practice, you could integrate Salute to the Sun into any of the other yoga practices in this book.

You could start or end this Winter Solstice Salute to the Sun with either Solar-Powered Breathing or the Four-Minute Check-in Meditation, which follow.

### Winter Solstice Yoga Practice Overview

1. Mountain Pose with Sun Visualization. Picture the sun rising in the sky. Picture a warm, glowing sun at solar plexus.

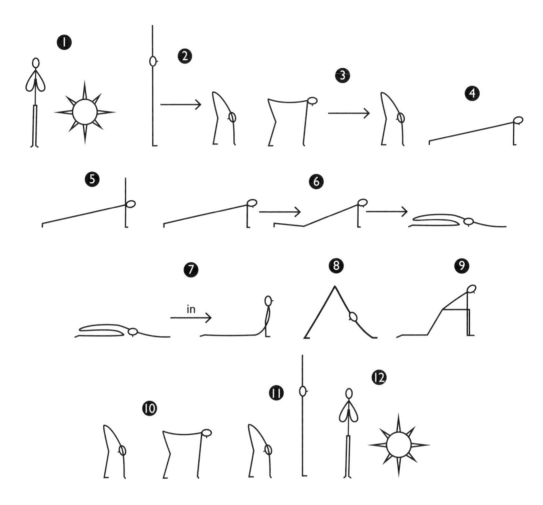

2. Raise arms above head and come into Standing Forward Bend.

3. Bend knees and arch back, and then come back down into Standing Forward Bend.

4. Step back into Plank Pose, with the whole body in one long line.

5. Swivel into Side Plank. Repeat on other side.

6. Plank Pose. Drop knees to floor and sit back into Child's Pose.

7. Child's Pose into Upward-Facing Dog.

8. Downward-Facing Dog. Stay a few breaths.

9. Bring foot forward into Lunge Pose.

10. Bring other foot forward into Standing Forward Bend, and then dip the back.

11. Standing Forward Bend. Stay for a few breaths. Standing up, sweep arms out to side and above head.

12. Mountain Pose with Sun Visualization. Rest here for a few breaths. Picture a warm, glowing sun at solar plexus and keep image in mind as you perform another round.

EXERCISE

## Solar-Powered Breathing

At the Winter Solstice, Solar-Powered Breathing brings warmth and sunshine into cold winter days. It can also be used at any other time of year to energize and recharge your batteries.

Solar-Powered Breathing will lift a low mood and create a sunnier outlook. If hormonal swings have left you feeling emotional, it will induce a sense of sunny optimism and vitality.

This breathing practice can be done lying, sitting, or standing. It can also be used when you hold a yoga pose, imagining that there is a warm sun at your solar plexus radiating rays of sunshine around your body.

Find yourself a comfortable position, either sitting, standing, or lying. Imagine that it is a warm, sunny summer's day. Picture the sun in the sky and feel the warmth of the sun on your skin.

Now imagine that you can locate the sun within your own body. Picture a sun radiating warmth, light, and energy at your solar plexus. If you wish, place your hands on your solar plexus (the area below your breastbone but above your navel).

Imagine that as you inhale you are breathing into the sun at your solar plexus, and as you exhale you are breathing out from there. Repeat for a few breaths.

Now imagine that with each inhale the sun is charged up, and on each exhale the sun expands and glows a little brighter.

**Inhale:** charge up

**Exhale:** expand

After a few breaths of breathing in this way, begin to send the sun's healing rays of energy all around the body. With each inhale the sun is recharged, and with each exhale the sun is radiating healing rays of light all around the body.

**Inhale:** recharge

**Exhale:** radiate

After a few breaths, go back to your normal breathing. Let go of the image of the sun at your solar plexus. Once again imagine that it is a warm, sunny summer's day. Picture the sun in the sky and feel the warmth of the sun on your skin.

Now let go of the image of the sunny day and bring your awareness back to your body; notice where your body is in contact with the floor or support. Notice how you are feeling and how you have been affected by the Solar-Powered Breathing. Resolve to take these warm, sunny feelings into your everyday life and the next thing that you do today.

EXERCISE

# The Four-Minute Check-In Meditation

The Four-Minute Check-In Meditation is a mindfulness-based meditation that once learnt can be a lifeline in so many situations.[24] It can be particularly useful during the hectic winter festivities, which can be a time when you most need meditation but seem to have zero time to devote to it. It can also be used all year round, whenever you need to settle and steady yourself.

This mini meditation will give support whenever you feel worried, anxious, stressed, unsettled, panicky, or overwhelmed. It only takes a few minutes to do and will help steady you so that you feel more able to cope with whatever situation arises.

If you can find a few minutes to spend on this meditation, it will actually save you time, as it restores a sense of perspective, preventing you from running around like the proverbial headless chicken. If you put in the time to learn and practice this meditation regularly, it will be there for you when you need it most, helping restore a sense of calm.

---

24. The Four-Minute Check-In Meditation is my interpretation of a popular mindfulness meditation called the Three Minute Breathing Space (you can find a free download of the Three Minute Breathing Space meditation on this website: franticworld.com/free-meditations-from-mindfulness).

This meditation can be done anywhere and anytime. Usually it is done standing, although it could be adapted to sitting or lying down. A simple way of remembering the four stages of the meditation is by the acronym SAGE: **s**tand tall, **a**wareness, **g**athering, **e**xpanding.

**Step 1: Stand Tall.** Assume an upright and dignified posture.

**Step 2: Awareness.** Become aware of any thoughts and feelings that are arising. Notice any bodily sensations that you are experiencing. Just observe your inner experience, without judging, shaping, or trying to change it.

**Step 3: Gathering.** Bring your awareness to your breathing. Notice how with each in- and out-breath the belly gently rises and falls. If your mind wanders off, gently bring it back to an awareness of the belly rising and falling with each breath.

**Step 4: Expanding Your Awareness.** Be aware of the breath at the belly and be aware of the whole body breathing. If any part of your body feels tight or tense, imagine that you are breathing into it on the in-breath and breathing out from it on the out-breath, softening, releasing, and letting go with each exhale. Allow your experience to be just as it is in this moment.

Resolve to take this more open, spacious, and accepting awareness into the next thing that you do today.

## Tree Wisdom in Winter

Spending time around trees is the perfect way to connect to the importance nature places upon conserving energy and resting during this cold, dark winter period.

When you are out and about, stop and spend some time mindfully observing a tree bare of all its leaves. Notice the shape the bare tree forms. Notice the space around the tree and the sky above it.

Do the same mindful observations with an evergreen tree.

As you do this mindfulness exercise, notice how you are feeling, what you are thinking, how your body is feeling, and the rhythm of your natural breath. If you are feeling cold, notice how it feels to be cold. If you are feeling snug and warm in your winter gear, notice how that feels too.

_____ EXERCISE _____
# Trees and Creativity during Winter

You can use the time that you have spent mindfully around trees as a springboard for your creativity. If you are stuck for ideas, here are a few to get you going:

- Mindfully draw a pencil sketch of a tree bare of leaves. You can draw either from observation or from memory.

- Track down some winter art to inspire you: paintings, songs, poems, stories, or photographs.

- Spend a few minutes considering how it feels to be a tree in winter. And then respond creatively to this question by writing, drawing, or singing or in any other way you choose.

- Find out more about the science behind how a tree conserves its energy and rests over the winter. Use the resources available to you online, in books, from a knowledgeable friend, and so on to find out more. Once you have done this, observe whether your newfound knowledge adds to or detracts from your enjoyment and appreciation of trees. Share your knowledge with friends.

## Meditation upon a Holly Tree at Winter Solstice

Last December, while doing research for this book, I headed up into the hills in pursuit of some ancient holly trees. With a bitingly cold wind blowing against me, I walked for a few miles uphill and eventually found an ancient grove of holly trees. The winter landscape was gray and bleak, but there was something exuberant and joyful about these holly trees growing on the hillside. Their old, curved, and contorted branches made them look like they were striking a pose and dancing. Their shiny, prickly green leaves and red berries caught the light and gave them a luminescent, spiritual feel. And young slender branches were growing out of the old wood.

The holly tree has taught me to dance through the seasons and to stay connected to my joy even on the darkest and coldest of winter days. It was mindfully spending time with these holly trees that inspired the tree prose poem below.

*The holly and the ivy dance through the sparkling streets, leading the*
*old solar year into the new. The Yuletide moon, a flower with four*

*white petals, smiles down upon the blood-of-life red holly, stealing*
*Xmas kisses, in darkened doorways, from white mistletoe.*

*O joyous good omen! Evergreen, when all the other trees have*
*lost their leaves. The holly is a dancer, a prancer, a leaper, and a*
*lover. Her leaves, a thousand mirrors, reflect the dilute winter*
*sunshine, and her scarlet berries sing songs of praise. Ding*
*dong merrily on high, in heaven the bells are ringing.*

*Flaming yellow gorse and red holly berries illuminate the*
*winter gloom. Fire in her spirit, the ancient holly tree is*
*dancing upon the mountain. New life in the midst of darkness,*
*her ancient trunk splits asunder and gives birth to slender new*
*branches, leaves prickly and green. Her red berries harvest the*
*fullness of the moon. And still I rise, and still I rise, she sings.*
*Of all the trees that are in the wood the holly bears the crown.*

## Winter Solstice Meditation Questions

These questions are designed to be used around the time of the winter solstice. It's fine to use them a week or two before or after the actual date of the solstice. Guidance on how to use the seasonal meditation questions can be found in chapter 1.

- In these dark days of winter who brings warmth and sunshine into my life?
  - How will I show them my gratitude?
  - What actions can I take to bring warmth and light into the lives of those who are close to me?

- Looking back over the past half year, since the summer solstice, what have I been incubating during this darker half of the year?
  - What have I learnt and what wisdom will I be taking with me into the New Year?
  - What will my spiritual focus be for the year ahead?

- The sun is reborn at the winter solstice. What is being reborn in me at this time?
  - ↬ What are my hopes and dreams for the coming year?
  - ↬ What do I want to achieve during the growing season?
  - ↬ Which projects do I wish to prioritize to make best use of the expansive energy of this lighter half of the year?
  - ↬ What am I passionate about? What lights my fire?
  - ↬ What actions will I need to take in the coming months to make my dreams manifest?
  - ↬ How will I stay in touch with my inner wisdom while taking action in the world?

- What do I wish to leave behind in the old year?
  - ↬ What do I need to sweep away to make room for the new?
  - ↬ What do I need to let go of to realize my dreams?

- How will I best look after myself over the winter and so avoid getting physically rundown or succumbing to the winter blues?
  - ↬ Which yoga practices could I use to reenergize and uplift me?
  - ↬ What other activities boost my mood?
  - ↬ Who brings a smile to my face and how will I go about connecting with them?

- At a time of year when overconsumption and overspending are encouraged, how can I make gift choices that are kind to the earth and don't use up precious resources?
  - ↬ Who would appreciate being given the gift of my time?
  - ↬ Who can I affirm and show how much I appreciate them?
  - ↬ Can I give the gift of really listening to someone and being *present* for them?
  - ↬ How do I ensure that whatever I choose to give is given with love?

- How will I connect with nature and appreciate the beauty of the season?

# CHAPTER NINE

# Winter Turns to Spring

*End of January to mid-March in the Northern Hemisphere*
*End of July to mid-September in the Southern Hemisphere*

The light is expanding, and the earth is awakening, bringing transformation, regeneration, and renewal. Use the solar energy of the season to fire up your intention to initiate change. Let go of the old to make room for the new. This is a time of new beginnings.

## Shaking Off Winter and Waking Up to Spring

The new growth cycle has begun, and although we haven't quite shaken off winter, there are signs that spring is on the way. The first lambs are gamboling in the field, the sun is shining on frostbitten grass, and green shoots are peeping up through the snow.

Between now and the summer solstice in June (December in the Southern Hemisphere), the light will be expanding. The sun is in its waxing phase, and this means that the direction of energy is moving from moon to sun, dark to light, water to fire, yin to yang, inner to outer, and from contemplation to action. Whatever seeds are planted now will expand and grow.

Over the coming weeks the year will rev up, and we too prepare to rev up our own energy so that we can make the most of this expansive, fertile growing season energy.

Gradually, we make a shift from inward reflection toward taking outward action. We also consider how we'll stay connected to our inner wisdom while acting in the world. The world is waking up after her winter sleep; new green shoots appear, flowers open, and blossom buds are forming on trees. In our own life we notice green shoots too, and we ask, what do we wish to blossom in our life over the coming months?

In theory, at this time we should be poised like an athlete at the starting line of a race, ready to leap into action. However, at the end of winter many of us are still in hibernation mode. Fortunately, our yoga practice can energize and help us shake off winter lethargy. We can take our lead from Nature; slowly she begins to paint jewellike splashes of color, life, and light into the monochrome winter landscapes. We too can make a slow transition, from the inward, contemplative focus of winter to the outward, active focus of spring.

The irrepressible creativity of nature is stirring as spring approaches. What is waking up inside of you at this time and wishing to be expressed? What is new within you and waiting to be brought out into the light? The waxing sun ignites a spark of passion within us and our ideas bloom like flowers.

Many studies show that creativity is good for your health and a great way of relaxing.[25] Your yoga and meditation practice can enhance your creativity by unlocking the treasure trove of your subconscious mind. Now is the time to get out that mindful coloring book and crayons that have been gathering dust on a high shelf, pick up that half-knitted jumper, bake an exquisite cake, make your body into a love song, dance a dance, paint a room, write a poem, design a yoga practice—just do whatever it takes to get your creative juices flowing.

We are at the tail end of winter, and soon the longer, warmer days will be with us again. Now is the time to talk with your loved ones about the things you want to do together this spring and summer. Have fun and make a love-to-do list; let your imagination run wild and come up with a list of fun activities for the coming months. And remember: magic happens!

During the growing season, whatever is planted will expand and grow, so now is the time to plant seeds of love. Relationships are like plants: they need to be nurtured and

---

25. Cathy Malchiodi, "Creativity as a Wellness Practice," Psychology Today, December 31, 2015, https://www.psychologytoday.com/blog/arts-and-health/201512/creativity-wellness-practice.

fed if they are to grow strong and flourish. Love is a garden, and if you take the time to feed and water your relationships, then love will blossom and grow.

## Getting Your Year into Gear!

Spring is a time of new beginnings. Now is a good time to review all aspects of your life and consider what changes you want to make. Research shows that we are more likely to make changes in our life if we talk beforehand about the changes we wish to make.[26] So, whether you want to go the gym more often, take up yoga, quit smoking, or eat more healthily, you have more chance of succeeding if you talk to friends, family, and colleagues about what you want to achieve first. This is called change talk. Change talk is when you acknowledge that there are obstacles that stand between you and your goal, and you talk to others about how you will overcome those obstacles. Change talk is motivating, and it means you gather around yourself a band of people to cheer you on to a healthier, happier lifestyle.

As the sun gets stronger, now is the time to fire up your dreams! If you are ambivalent about swinging into action, that's natural. Just remember to pace yourself. A good way to make the transition from contemplation to action is to allow your action to be guided by your inner wisdom. Your yoga practice can help you to stay centered and grounded, enabling you not to get swept away by the speed, activity, and rush of the coming growing season energy.

What should we do if our dreams have stalled? Sometimes when we feel stuck, it helps to take baby steps, in order to start moving forward again. Or, if you're staring at a blank page not knowing what to write, just jot down a few words: make a start and more ideas will follow. Baby steps get you moving, get your energy flowing, and prevent stagnation. Take another look at what you want to achieve this growing season, and then break this down into smaller, manageable steps. Which of these is the smallest, easiest step you could take? Resolve to take that step! Now you're moving forward again.

The ritual of spring cleaning is a gentle way of transitioning from an inward focus to taking action. Completing a mundane job such as tidying your desk or cleaning out a cupboard can shift stuck energy, lift your mood, and boost your confidence. Spring cleaning brushes away the cobwebs and stagnant energy that has collected over winter.

---

26. Hal Arkowitz, Henny A. Westra, William R. Miller, and Stephen Rollnick, eds., *Motivational Interviewing in the Treatment of Psychological Problems* (New York: The Guilford Press, 2008), 8, 16, 17, 337.

If done mindfully, cleaning can be a meditation. (Remember to get your housemates to share in the joy of this housework meditation so that it doesn't end up becoming a chore.)

If you're feeling run-down at the end of winter, you might feel the need to give yourself a good spring clean and detox. This makes it a good time to look at the yogic approach to purity (*sauca*), which is one of the observances, or the personal disciplines, that make up the second of Patanjali's eight limbs of yoga.

Yoga practice does undeniably have a beneficial purifying and cleansing effect on our system. Yoga postures, breathing practices, meditation, and relaxation all help us let go and detoxify, on both a mental and physical level. However, it's important to make sure that self-discipline doesn't turn into an unhealthy self-denial of enjoyment of all the good things in life. Moderation in all things, including moderation!

In the world today, there is money to be made from making people (women in particular) feel "impure" and bad about themselves. Our yoga practice can provide a great antidote to this, as it teaches us to focus on how we feel on the inside, rather than obsessing about our outward appearance. Which yoga techniques have you found help you to access a sense of being okay as you are? What else has helped you feel comfortable in your own skin and good about yourself?

If we do find ourselves striving to create a bubble of purity, it's worth widening the lens and shifting our focus from our own individual purification to working to create a world that is pure and unpolluted for everyone to enjoy. What small steps could you take to make this dream a reality? The intense beauty of the earth in spring reminds us of the need to take care of this precious planet that we call home.

## Growing Your Own Home Yoga Practice

Early spring is a great time to get creative with your yoga practice. Seeds planted now will expand and grow, so why not spend some time and energy planting out seeds for a dazzling yoga garden?

There are many advantages to having a home yoga practice:

- It's quality time for you. It's tailored to meet your needs; you can strengthen and tone or relax and unwind.
- It is a healing space where you can nurture and nourish yourself.

- It frees up your creativity and leaves you feeling inspired.

- It's free—no expensive gym membership.

- It's enjoyable, and portable too. Wherever you go, your yoga goes with you! With all these benefits, why wouldn't you practice yoga at home?

At the end of winter your home yoga practice might need some freshening up. Or perhaps you want to practice yoga at home but don't yet have the confidence. Or your home practice has lapsed, and you want to start it up again. Or maybe you are a yoga teacher suffering from burn-out. Whatever your reasons, here are some questions that will help you kick-start your home yoga practice:

- What would the benefits of doing a regular home yoga practice be?

- What are the obstacles that stand in the way of practicing yoga at home?

- How will I overcome these obstacles? Which one would be the easiest to tackle?

- If everything went well and I managed to establish a regular home yoga practice, what would it look like? What would I be doing? How would I be feeling? How would my life be different from how it is now?

I have always had a yoga home practice. This is partly due to circumstances, as when I started yoga in my early teens, I wasn't old enough to go to classes. While waiting for my sixteenth birthday to arrive so I could enroll in a class, I taught myself from books and magazines at home. During this time, yoga became such a personal thing to me that when I did eventually get to my first yoga class, it felt odd to be practicing yoga with other people, a bit like finding yourself naked in a public place! My favorite experience of yoga is still doing it myself at home, and my best teachers are books.

What I try to convey and channel through my teaching is the sense of peace and joy that I derive from my own yoga practice. My intention when I teach is to create an atmosphere where my students can blossom and unfold. I want them to access a peaceful, nourishing, nurturing space within, just as I do myself in my own practice. My home yoga practice is like a deep well that I can draw on to nourish myself and to fuel my teaching.

Initially, it might feel scary to step onto your yoga mat, with just your thoughts, feelings, and bodily sensations for company. It takes courage to come face to face with your true self in yoga. In my younger days I had debilitating anxiety, and being confronted with anxious thoughts during my yoga practice often felt overwhelming. However, over the years I have learnt that if you can stay present to uncomfortable thoughts and feelings as they arise, you uncover within yourself a peaceful place that can lovingly hold and contain them. If you persevere, you will discover within this "aloneness" a sense of freedom, connection, and healing.

A good way to start a home practice is to commit to a daily practice of five to ten minutes a day. Once you are in this habit, you'll find that you feel so good from doing it that you want to do more. A little forward planning goes a long way; spend some time working out what your practice will be before you step onto your mat. Or, if you feel confident enough, step onto your mat and see where your inner wisdom leads you!

A good way of building confidence and getting used to spending time on your own doing yoga might be to start off using a yoga DVD or YouTube video. To create a calming ambience, light a candle or put on some relaxing music on. All these small steps are ways of planting the seeds of an established yoga practice, and before you know it, your yoga garden will be in full bloom!

## Winter to Spring Yoga Practice

As winter turns to spring the world is waking up and coming back to life again. This yoga practice is inspired by the first spring flowers opening into blossom, heralding the arrival of spring.

The practice incorporates a theme of opening and closing to encapsulate that end-of-winter feeling and coming out of hibernation. The yoga flow from Child's Pose to Upward-Facing Dog reflects this sense of waking up to spring after a long winter sleep.

The practice is energizing and revitalizing. It will help you shake off winter lethargy, boost your mood, and banish winter blues. It opens you up to new possibilities.

It can also be used at any other time of the year. Allow 15 to 20 minutes

### 1. Blossoming Hands

Close your eyes and draw your awareness inward (or if you prefer, keep your eyes open). Begin to gently open and close your fingers. Make a gentle fist, like a flower closing back to bud. Then spread the fingers like a flower opening. Continue to slowly and gently repeat this opening and closing movement.

Once you have established a rhythm to the movement, bring your awareness to the natural flow of your breath. As you observe the breath, notice how it corresponds to the opening and closing movement of the hands. More detailed instructions for this exercise can be found after this yoga practice.

Blossoming Hands

## 2. Flower Arms

Stand tall, feet hip width apart. In your mind's eye picture your favorite spring flower. Now place fingertips on shoulders, elbows out to the side; relax shoulders down away from ears. Inhale and open arms out to the side, like a flower opening. Exhale and bend arms, bringing fingertips back to shoulders, like a flower closing back to bud. Repeat 6 times.

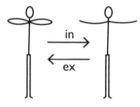

Flower Arms

## 3. Albatross Sequence 2

Stand tall, feet hip width apart, hands resting on your belly. Inhale and raise arms. Exhale and sweep the arms out to the sides like a bird's wings as you bend halfway forward, back slightly arched, into Albatross Pose. Stay here and inhale. Exhale and lower into Standing Forward Bend (*Uttanasana*). Inhale, bending the knees and arching the back. Exhale back down into Forward Bend. Inhale and sweep arms out to the side and up above the head as you come back up to standing. Exhale and lower the hands back to belly. Repeat the sequence 4 times. (See Summer to Autumn Yoga Practice on page 82 for Albatross Sequence 1.)

*For a shorter practice, finish here.*

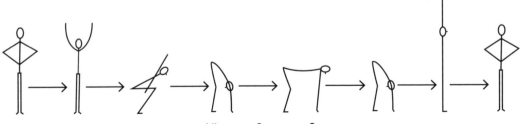

Albatross Sequence 2

### 4. Warrior 2 Pose (*Virabhadrasana 2*)

Take the legs wide apart; left foot turns slightly in and right foot turns out. Bend the right knee. Take the arms out at shoulder height, palms facing down. Turn your head to look along your right arm. Stay here for a few breaths. Repeat on the other side.

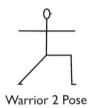

Warrior 2 Pose

### 5. Wide-Leg Standing Forward Bend Pose (*Prasarita Padottanasana*)

Take the legs wide apart, feet parallel. Raise the arms out to the sides, just below shoulder height. Inhale and hinge forward from the hip joints into a wide-leg forward bend. Bring the hands to the floor (or for a gentler option, bring the hands to rest on the legs or on raised blocks). Stay here for a few breaths. Return to the starting position.

Wide-Leg Standing Forward Bend Pose

### 6. Lunge Pose (*Anjaneyasana*) into Hamstring Stretch

Come to tall kneeling. Take your right foot forward; bend the right knee over the ankle. Take your hands to the heart in the Prayer Position (*Namaste*). For a gentler option, keep the hands here or raise the arms above the head. Stay here for a few breaths. Then come into Hamstring Stretch by straightening the front, right leg, leaning the torso forward over the leg, and resting your fingertips on the floor on either side of the front leg. Stay for a few breaths and then repeat on the other side.

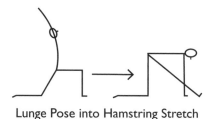

Lunge Pose into Hamstring Stretch

### 7. Downward-Facing Dog Pose (*Adho Mukha Svanasana*)

Come onto all fours; turn the toes under and push up into Downward Facing Dog Pose (*Adho Mukha Svanasana*). Stay here for a few breaths.

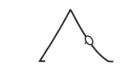

Downward-Facing Dog Pose

### 8. Child's Pose (*Balasana*) into Upward-Facing Dog (*Urdhva Mukha Svanasana*)

From Downward-Facing Dog bend the knees and sit back into Child's Pose (*Balasana*), arms outstretched along the floor. From Child's Pose inhale and move forward into Upward-Facing Dog (*Urdhva Mukha Svanasana*), arching your back and keeping your knees on the floor. Exhale back into Child's Pose. Repeat 6 times.

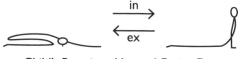

Child's Pose into Upward-Facing Dog

### 9. Bridge Pose (*Setu Bandhasana*) into Knees-to-Chest Pose (*Apanasana*)

Lie on your back, knees bent, feet on the floor hip width apart, arms by your sides. Inhale and peel your back from the floor, taking your arms overhead onto the floor behind you, coming into Bridge Pose. Exhale and lower the back, returning the arms to the sides. Still exhaling (or take an extra breath), curl up into a ball; bring the knees to the chest and the hands to the knees, into Knees-to-Chest Pose. Inhale and come back to the starting position. Stay for one breath and then repeat the sequence. Repeat 4 to 6 times.

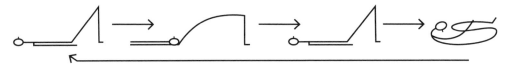

Bridge Pose into Knees-to-Chest Pose

### 10. Knees-to-Chest Pose (*Apanasana*) into Wide-Leg Stretch

Bring the knees into the chest; rest the fingertips lightly on the knees. Inhale and take the arms overhead and straighten the legs up vertically, heels toward the ceiling. Exhale and take the legs out into a wide V shape. Inhale and bring the legs together again. Exhale and bend the knees into the chest, bringing the fingertips back to the knees. Repeat sequence 4 to 6 times.

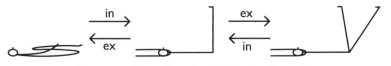

Knees-to-Chest Pose into Wide-Leg Stretch

### 11. Blossoming Hands

Rest for a few breaths here, with knees bent and feet on the floor. Close your eyes and draw your awareness inward (or if you prefer, keep your eyes open). Begin to gently open and close your fingers. Make a gentle fist, like a flower closing back to bud. Then spread the fingers, like a flower opening. Continue to slowly and gently repeat this opening and closing movement.

Once you have established a rhythm to the movement, bring your awareness to the natural flow of your breath. As you observe the breath, notice how it corresponds to the opening and closing movement of the hands. More detailed instructions for this exercise can be found on page 161.

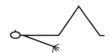

Blossoming Hands

## Winter to Spring Yoga Practice Overview

1. Blossoming Hands. Gently open and close fingers. Make a gentle fist, like a flower closing back to bud. Then spread fingers, like a flower opening. Notice how the breath corresponds to opening and closing movement of hands.

2. Flower Arms. Stand tall, feet hip width apart. Picture your favorite spring flower. Inhale: open arms out to the side, like a flower opening. Exhale: bend arms, bringing finger tips back to shoulders, like a flower closing back to bud. Repeat × 6.

3. Albatross Sequence 2. Repeat × 4.

4. Warrior 2. Stay for a few breaths. Repeat on other side.

5. Wide-Leg Standing Forward Bend. Stay for a few breaths.

6. Lunge Pose into Hamstring Stretch. Stay for a few breaths. Repeat on other side.

7. Downward-Facing Dog. Stay for a few breaths.

8. Child's Pose into Upward-Facing Dog. Repeat × 6.

9. Bridge Pose into Knees-to-Chest Pose. Inhale: into Bridge Pose. Exhale: lower the back, returning arms to sides. Still exhaling (or take extra breath) curl up into Knees-to-Chest Pose. Inhale back to the starting position. Stay for one breath. Repeat × 4–6.

10. Knees-to-Chest into Wide-Leg Stretch. Repeat × 4–6.

11. Blossoming Hands. Gently open and close fingers. Make a gentle fist, like a flower closing back to bud. Then spread fingers, like a flower opening. Notice how the breath corresponds to opening and closing movement of hands.

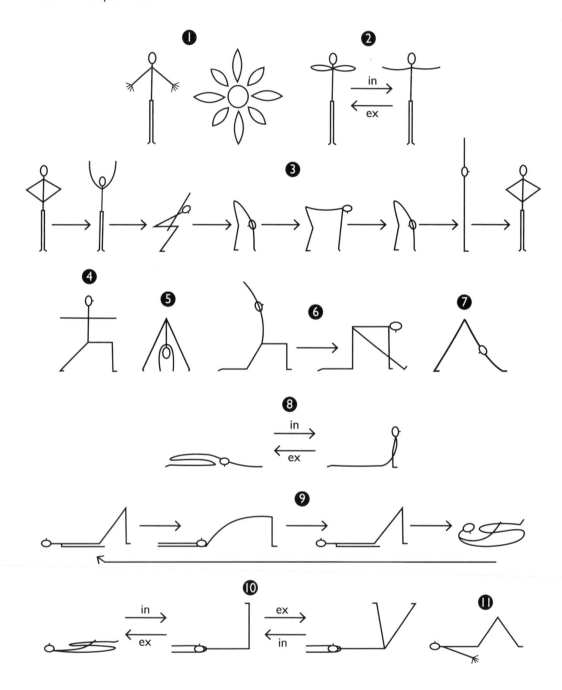

# Blossoming Hands

The Blossoming Hands exercise frees up the breathing, establishing a healthy, relaxed breathing pattern. It also helps maintain suppleness and flexibility of the hands. It has a subtle opening effect on the body's posture and helps gently energize and lift the mood.

It's a great way to start a yoga practice. The practice could then be themed around the idea of opening and closing. It can also be used anytime as a stand-alone practice.

Find yourself a comfortable position, either standing, sitting, or lying down. If you are standing, stand with your arms by your side and palms facing forward. If you are sitting, sit with your palms facing up and resting on your thighs. If you are lying down, have both knees bent, feet on the floor and about hip width apart. Arms are by your sides with the palms facing up.

Close your eyes and draw your awareness inward (or if you prefer, keep the eyes open). Begin to gently open and close your fingers. Make a gentle fist, like a flower closing back to bud. Then spread the fingers, like a flower opening. Continue to slowly and gently repeat this opening and closing movement. Once you have established a rhythm to the movement, bring your awareness to the flow of your breath. Breathe naturally; do not try to control the breath.

As you observe the breath, notice in what way the breath corresponds to the opening and closing movement of the hands. Notice when you are breathing in or out in relation to the movement. Simply observe what's happening as you breathe and move. There's no right or wrong way to do it.

When you feel ready, gradually allow the movement to subside and come to rest. Continue to observe the flow of your breath and notice what effect the blossoming hands exercise has had upon you.

## Tree Wisdom in Winter to Spring

When you are out and about, be on the lookout for signs of fresh growth and new life appearing on trees, such as blossom or leaf buds. Also see if you can notice signs of life around the tree, such as spring flowers, birds, or small animals. Use all your senses to mindfully enjoy these signs that nature is coming back to life again.

EXERCISE
_____

## Trees and Creativity
## during Winter to Spring

You can use the time that you have spent mindfully with trees as a springboard for your creativity. If you are stuck for ideas, here are a few ideas to get you started:

- Take some photos on the theme of *signs of the arrival of spring*. Use them as screen savers. Or print them out and pin them up in places where they will inspire and uplift you. Or share them on social media to cheer and inspire others.

- If you have a favorite type of tree, find out any myths and stories associated with it. Or make up your own myth!

- If you feel an affinity with a particular tree, spend a few moments imagining what this tree would say if it could talk. If you wish, use this tree monologue to inspire your creativity, in whatever medium that appeals to you.

- Grow something! Even if you don't have a garden, you can grow things indoors, such as cress on cotton wool or a potted avocado stone. Or find out if you can join in with tree planting in your area.

- Try out this chapter's Winter to Spring Yoga Practice, inspired by a blossom opening in spring.

### Meditation upon a Rowan Tree in Winter to Spring

In the center of my garden grows a rowan tree, encircled by a hexagonal wooden table, built for us by a carpenter friend. Every year during the winter the tree is laden down with orange berries, which the birds love to feast upon. According to myth, the rowan tree offers protection when it is planted near the house. Rowan is considered to be a magical tree because on each berry there is to be found a star-shaped pentacle, which is a magical symbol. The rowan tree is known as a flying tree because it sometimes grows almost horizontally from the sides of mountains, and its leaves look like eagles' wings.

The rowan tree has taught me how to create an extraordinary, magical gift out of ordinary, everyday ingredients—and to keep on giving that gift the whole year round. It was mindfully spending time around rowan trees that inspired this tree prose poem:

*I am the Rowan Tree, rainbow tree of immortality, ambrosia to the gods. Slender gray bough; leaves green, pink, gold, and branches reaching up to the heavens. My roots in the soil, wrapping around rocks; my eagle wings take flight and alight where mountainside meets sky. Magical tree, a five-pointed star on each scarlet berry; I offer you protection when I grow near your home. Five petals, five sepals, my creamy-white blossom is the milk of human kindness. I am your mother, daughter, sister, and friend. Creativity, my wood is the spinning wheel that spins the thread of life. Generosity, the lifeblood of fertility, fire in the belly; the first woman was born from a rowan tree.*

## Winter to Spring Meditation Questions

These questions are designed to be used any time from around the end of January to mid-February in the Northern Hemisphere and from around the end of July to mid-August in the Southern Hemisphere. Guidance on how to use the seasonal meditation questions can be found in chapter 1.

- Nature is coming back to life after her winter sleep. What signs have I noticed of green shoots in my life?

- This is the start of the growing season; whatever is set in motion now will expand and grow. What do I wish to grow more of in my life?
    - ↬ Which projects do I wish to prioritize, in order that they might have the best chance of coming to fruition over the next few months?
    - ↬ What actions will I need to take to ensure a successful outcome?
    - ↬ How can I connect and collaborate with others to ensure the success of each venture?

- What will my spiritual focus for the year be?
    - ↬ Which values will guide my actions over the coming months?
    - ↬ How will I stay in touch with my inner wisdom while taking outward action?

- What do I wish to grow in my relationships? What are the seeds of love that I will be planting out?
  - ↬ What loving actions could I take to ensure my relationships grow healthy and strong?

- Traditionally, this is a time for spring cleaning. Are there any areas of my life that would benefit from a good spring clean?
  - ↬ Does my work or home environment need a good clean to clear out stagnant energy?
  - ↬ What physical clutter can I let go of?

- Are there any steps I can take, big or small, to make the earth's environment cleaner and healthier?

- In spring Nature is at her most creative. How can I draw inspiration from the natural world and allow my own creativity to blossom?
  - ↬ Can I channel some of this spring-inspired creativity into designing imaginative and nourishing yoga practices for myself?
  - ↬ Are there any blocks to my creative expression? How will I go about removing them?

- Between now and the summer solstice the days will get longer and the sun stronger. Where is the fiery passion in my life?
  - ↬ Which activities will nurture and nourish me?
  - ↬ Which activities are depleting or unhelpful and how do I reduce these?
  - ↬ How can I have fun? What do I enjoy doing? What am I passionate about? What lights my fire? What makes me happy?

- Are there any seeds of positivity that I could plant to help the various communities that I am a part of to grow healthy and strong?

- As new life unfolds and the first signs of spring appear, what are my plans for getting out and about to enjoy the beauty of the season?

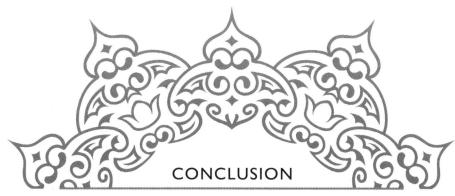

CONCLUSION

# Every Ending
# Is a New Beginning

*Spring, summer, autumn, winter… and spring comes around again.*

The Seasonal Yoga journey is a circular one. Throughout the seasons and across the years this book is here for you to dip into for seasonal guidance and inspiration. As you gain experience of working in harmony with the seasons, I hope that you will make Seasonal Yoga your own in a creative and joyful way.

Each of us can reinvent and reimagine yoga in a way that is inclusive and respectful to all genders and the earth. If you can find the courage to share your reimagined yoga with others, we will all be the richer for it. This book is my gift to you, *my* authentic experience and reimagining of yoga.

At the start of the book we remembered that legend has it that yoga was born from the womb of the earth. When we connect with the earth through our seasonal practice, we are united with yoga itself.

I hope that your exploration helps you feel a deep connection to the sun, the moon, the earth, and yourself. And may this connection allow you to access a deep source of energy and wisdom that empowers you to act in a loving, compassionate, and caring way to yourself, your fellow travelers, and this beautiful planet that spins us through the seasons.

# Bibliography

Achterberg, Jeanne. *Woman as Healer: A Comprehensive Survey from Prehistoric Times to the Present Day*. London: Random Century Group, 1990.

Arkowitz, Hal, Henny A. Westra, William R. Miller, and Stephen Rollnick, eds. *Motivational Interviewing in the Treatment of Psychological Problems*. New York: The Guilford Press, 2008.

Barrett, Ruth. *Women's Rites, Women's Mysteries: Intuitive Ritual Creation*. Woodbury, MN: Llewellyn Publications, 2007. Pages 177–210.

Cameron, Julia. *The Artist's Way: A Course in Discovering and Recovering Your Creative Self*. London: Pan Books, 1995.

De Michelis, Elizabeth. *A History of Modern Yoga*. London: Continuum, 2005.

Denton, Lynn Teskey. *Female Ascetics in Hinduism*. Albany, NY: State University of New York Press, 2004.

Desikachar, T. K. V. *The Heart of Yoga: Developing Personal Practice*. Rochester, VT: Inner Traditions International, 1995.

Eliade, Mircea. *Yoga: Immortality and Freedom*. Princeton, NJ: Princeton University Press, 1958.

Feuerstein, Georg. *Encyclopedic Dictionary of Yoga*. London: Unwin Hyman, 1990.

———. *The Yoga Tradition: Its History, Literature, Philosophy and Practice.* Prescott, AZ: Hohm Press, 2001.

Gates, Janice. *Yogini: The Power of Women in Yoga.* San Rafael, CA: Mandala Publishing, 2006.

Germer, Christopher K. *The Mindful Path to Self-Compassion: Freeing Yourself from Destructive Thoughts and Emotions.* New York: The Guilford Press, 2009.

Gifford, Jane. *The Celtic Wisdom of Trees: Mysteries, Magic and Medicine.* London: Godsfield Press, 2000.

Goldberg, Natalie. *Writing Down the Bones: Freeing the Writer Within.* Boston, MA: Shambhala Publications, 1986.

Gordon, Amie M. "Gratitude Is for Lovers." Greater Good Magazine. February 5, 2013. https://greatergood.berkeley.edu/article/item/gratitude_is_for_lovers.

Griffin, Susan. *Woman and Nature: The Roaring Inside Her.* London: The Women's Press, 1984.

Gupta, Roxanne Kamayani. *A Yoga of Indian Classical Dance: The Yogini's Mirror.* Rochester, VT: Inner Traditions International, 2000.

Holmes, Jean. *Women in Religion.* With John Bowker. New York: Continuum, 2004. Pages 59–84.

Iyengar, B. K. S. *The Tree of Yoga.* London: Thorsons, 2000.

Kindred, Glennie. *The Alchemist's Journey: An Old System for a New Age.* London: Hay House Hay House UK, 2005.

———. *Earth Wisdom: A Heart-Warming Mixture of the Spiritual, the Practical, and the Proactive.* London: Hay House UK, 2004.

Knott, Kim. *Hinduism: A Very Short Introduction.* Oxford, UK: Oxford University Press, 2000.

Lasater, Judith. *Living Your Yoga: Finding the Spiritual in Everyday Life.* Berkeley, CA: Rodmell Press, 2000.

McDaniel, June. *Offering Flowers, Feeding Skulls: Popular Goddess Worship in West Bengal.* New York: Oxford University Press, 2004.

Mitchell, Stephen, trans. *Tao Te Ching: The Book of the Way.* London: Kyle Cathie, 2002.

Monk Kidd, Sue. *The Dance of the Dissident Daughter: A Woman's Journey from Christian Tradition to the Sacred Feminine.* New York: HarperCollins Publishers, 2002.

Nhat Hanh, Thich. *The Long Road Turns to Joy: A Guide to Walking Meditation.* Berkeley, CA: Parallax Press, 2011.

Orsillo, Susan M., and Lizabeth Roemer. *The Mindful Way through Anxiety: Break Free from Chronic Anxiety and Reclaim Your Life.* New York: The Guilford Press, 2011.

Pinkola Estés, Clarissa. *Women Who Run with the Wolves: Contacting the Power of the Wild Woman.* London: Random House, 1992.

Pintchman, Tracy, ed. *Women's Lives, Women's Rituals in the Hindu Tradition.* Oxford, UK: Oxford University Press, 2007.

Simmer-Brown, Judith. *Dakini's Warm Breath: The Feminine Principle in Tibetan Buddhism.* Boston, MA: Shambhala Publications, 2003.

Stoler Miller, Barbara. *Yoga: Discipline of Freedom; The Yoga Sutra Attributed to Patanjali.* New York: Bantam Books, 1998.

Stone, Merlin. *When God Was a Woman.* Orlando, FL: Harcourt Brace, 1976.

Walker, Alice. *We Are the Ones We Have Been Waiting For: Inner Light in a Time of Darkness.* London: Orion Publishing Group, 2007.

Walker, Barbara G. *The Woman's Dictionary of Symbols and Sacred Objects.* New York: HarperCollins Publishers, 1988.

———. *The Woman's Encyclopedia of Myths and Secrets.* New York: HarperCollins Publishers, 1983.

Wohlleben, Peter. *The Hidden Life of Trees: What They Feel, How They Communicate; Discoveries from a Secret World.* Vancouver, BC, Canada: Greystone Books, 2015.

# Recommended Resources

## Yoga Practice

Bennett, Bija. *Emotional Yoga: How the Body Can Heal the Mind.* London: Bantam Books, 2002.

Farhi, Donna. *Yoga Mind, Body & Spirit: A Return to Wholeness.* New York: Henry Holt Company, 2000.

Kraftsow, Gary. *Yoga for Transformation.* New York: Penguin Group, 2002.

———. *Yoga for Wellness: Healing with the Timeless Teachings of Viniyoga.* New York: Penguin Group, 1999.

Lee, Cyndi. *Yoga Body, Buddha Mind: A Complete Manual for Physical and Spiritual Well-Being from the Founder of the Om Yoga Center.* New York: Riverhead Books, 2004.

Powers, Sarah. *Insight Yoga: An Innovative Synthesis of Traditional Yoga, Meditation, and Eastern Approaches to Healing and Well-Being.* Boston, MA: Shambhala Publications, 2008.

Sabatini, Sandra. *Breath: The Essence of Yoga.* London: Thorsons, 2000.

Scaravelli, Vanda. *Awakening the Spine: The Stress-Free New Yoga That Works with the Body to Restore Health, Vitality, and Energy.* New York: HarperCollins Publishers, 1991.

## Yoga for Beginners

Lasater, Judith. *30 Essential Yoga Poses: For Beginning Students and Their Teachers.* Berkeley, CA: Rodmell Press, 2003.

Pierce, Margaret D., and Martin G. Pierce. *Yoga for Your Life: A Practice Manual of Breath and Movement.* Portland, OR: Rudra Press, 1996.

Rountree, Sage. *Everyday Yoga: At-Home Routines to Enhance Fitness, Build Strength, and Restore Your Body.* Boulder, CO: Velopress, 2015.

Esther Ekhart's wonderful website is an invaluable resource for beginners and more experienced students: www.ekhartyoga.com.

There are also lots of brilliant resources for beginners and more experienced students to be found on the Yoga Journal website: www.yogajournal.com.

## Mindfulness and Self-Compassion

Burch, Vidyamala, and Claire Irvin. *Mindfulness for Women: Declutter Your Mind, Simplify Your Life, Find Time to "Be."* London: Piatkus, 2016.

Gilbert, Paul. *The Compassionate Mind.* London: Constable & Robinson, 2009.

Neff, Kristin. *Self-Compassion: Stop Beating Yourself Up and Leave Insecurity Behind.* London: Hodder & Stoughton, 2011.

Nhat Hanh, Thich. *Mindful Movements: Ten Exercises for Well-Being.* Berkeley, CA: Parallax Press, 2008.

Orsillo, Susan M., and Lizabeth Roemer. *The Mindful Way through Anxiety: Break Free from Chronic Anxiety and Reclaim Your Life.* New York: The Guilford Press, 2011.

Williams, Mark, and Danny Penman. *Mindfulness: A Practical Guide to Finding Peace in a Frantic World.* London: Piatkus, 2011.

## To Write to the Author

If you wish to contact the author or would like more information about this book, please write to the author in care of Llewellyn Worldwide Ltd. and we will forward your request. Both the author and publisher appreciate hearing from you and learning of your enjoyment of this book and how it has helped you. Llewellyn Worldwide Ltd. cannot guarantee that every letter written to the author can be answered, but all will be forwarded. Please write to:

Jilly Shipway
℅ Llewellyn Worldwide
2143 Wooddale Drive
Woodbury, MN 55125-2989
Please enclose a self-addressed stamped envelope for reply,
or $1.00 to cover costs. If outside the U.S.A., enclose
an international postal reply coupon.

Many of Llewellyn's authors have websites with additional information and resources. For more information, please visit our website at http://www.llewellyn.com.

# GET MORE AT LLEWELLYN.COM

Visit us online to browse hundreds of our books and decks, plus sign up to receive our e-newsletters and exclusive online offers.

- Free tarot readings • Spell-a-Day • Moon phases
- Recipes, spells, and tips • Blogs • Encyclopedia
- Author interviews, articles, and upcoming events

# GET SOCIAL WITH LLEWELLYN

Find us on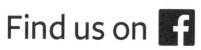

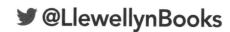 @LlewellynBooks

www.Facebook.com/LlewellynBooks

# GET BOOKS AT LLEWELLYN

## LLEWELLYN ORDERING INFORMATION

 **Order online:** Visit our website at www.llewellyn.com to select your books and place an order on our secure server.

 **Order by phone:**
- Call toll free within the US at 1-877-NEW-WRLD (1-877-639-9753)
- We accept VISA, MasterCard, American Express, and Discover.

 **Order by mail:**
Send the full price of your order (MN residents add 6.875% sales tax) in US funds plus postage and handling to: Llewellyn Worldwide, 2143 Wooddale Drive, Woodbury, MN 55125-2989

**POSTAGE AND HANDLING**

STANDARD (US):(Please allow 12 business days)
$30.00 and under, add $6.00.
$30.01 and over, FREE SHIPPING.

CANADA:
We cannot ship to Canada, please shop your local bookstore or Amazon Canada.

INTERNATIONAL:
Customers pay the actual shipping cost to the final destination, which includes tracking information.

Visit us online for more shipping options. Prices subject to change.

## FREE CATALOG!

To order, call
1-877-
NEW-WRLD
ext. 8236
or visit our
website

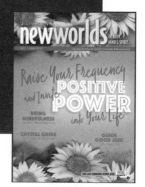

"Alanna has pioneered a relevant, educational book, deep thinking and laced with humor."
—Ana T. Forrest, founder of Forrest Yoga and author of *Fierce Medicine*

# yoga
## BEYOND THE MAT

HOW TO MAKE YOGA YOUR SPIRITUAL PRACTICE

ALANNA KAIVALYA, PhD

# Yoga Beyond the Mat
*How to Make Yoga Your Spiritual Practice*
ALANNA KAIVALYA, PHD

While many engage in asana, the physical practice, yoga's most transformative effects are found in the realms of the spiritual and psychological. *Yoga Beyond the Mat* shows you how to develop a personal, holistic yoga practice to achieve lasting and permanent transformation. Join Alanna Kaivalya as she guides you through a complete range of topics, including:

- Removing obstacles
- Appreciating the present moment
- Balancing the chakras
- Healing childhood wounds
- Creating your own rituals
- Transforming your archetypal energy
- Entering the blissful state

This book shows you that yoga doesn't make your life easier; it makes you better at your life. Through ritual, meditation, journaling, asana, and other spiritual practices, *Yoga Beyond the Mat* provides techniques for developing a personal mythology and allowing the ego to rest, leading modern-day yogis toward what they have been missing: the realization of personal bliss.

**978-0-7387-4764-4, 264 pp., 6 x 9**                                 **$16.99**

---

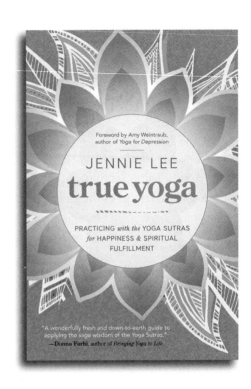

Foreword by Amy Weintraub,
author of *Yoga for Depression*

JENNIE LEE

true yoga

PRACTICING *with the* YOGA SUTRAS
*for* HAPPINESS & SPIRITUAL
FULFILLMENT

"A wonderfully fresh and down-to-earth guide to
applying the sage wisdom of the Yoga Sutras."
—**Donna Farhi**, author of *Bringing Yoga to Life*

# True Yoga
## *Practicing With the Yoga Sutras*
## *for Happiness & Spiritual Fulfillment*
### JENNIE LEE

Achieve lasting happiness no matter what life brings. *True Yoga* is an inspirational guide that shows you how to overcome difficulties and create sustainable joy through the Eight Limbs of Yoga outlined in the Yoga Sutras. Whether challenged by work, health, relationships, or parenting, you'll find tangible practices to illuminate your every day and spiritual life.

Using daily techniques, self-inquiry questions, and inspiring affirmations, yoga therapist Jennie Lee presents a system that opens the path to fulfillment and helps you connect with your own divinity. Discover effective methods for maintaining positive thoughts, managing stress, improving communication, and building new habits for success. By integrating the ancient wisdom of the Yoga Sutras into an accessible format, Lee puts the formula for enduring happiness within your reach.

**978-0-7387-4625-8, 264 pp., 5 ¼ x 8**                                    **$16.99**

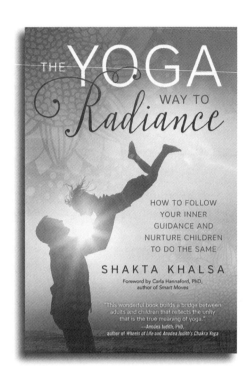

THE **YOGA**
WAY TO
*Radiance*

HOW TO FOLLOW
YOUR INNER
GUIDANCE AND
NURTURE CHILDREN
TO DO THE SAME

SHAKTA KHALSA

Foreword by Carla Hannaford, PhD,
author of *Smart Moves*

"This wonderful book builds a bridge between
adults and children that reflects the unity
that is the true meaning of yoga."
—Anodea Judith, PhD,
author of *Wheels of Life* and *Anodea Judith's Chakra Yoga*

# The Yoga Way to Radiance
*How to Follow Your Inner Guidance and Nurture Children to Do the Same*
SHAKTA KHALSA

Join author Shakta Khalsa on an experiential journey, exploring yoga-based tools to help you embrace your true self and live with wonder and joy as you care for the children in your life. *The Yoga Way to Radiance* has been written with the intention of helping you—whether you're a parent, family member, teacher, therapist, or caregiver—reclaim your authentic self while also helping the children around you stay connected to their own inner radiance. With Shakta's guidance, you'll discover:

- Fun, effective yoga exercises and meditations for children and adults
- Ancient wisdom and leading-edge teachings to help children be the radiant beings that they are
- Techniques for staying connected to your inner self while meeting challenges with children
- Tips for the art of deep listening and neutral, friendly talk
- Natural discipline that uses the magic of imagination and natural consequences
- How to place trust in a child's natural self-correcting abilities

**978-0-7387-4776-7, 216 pp., 6 x 9**                                           **$16.99**

# YOGA

*for the*

## Creative Soul

*Exploring the Five Paths of Yoga
to Reclaim Your Expressive Spirit*

## ERIN BYRON, MA

## Yoga for the Creative Soul
*Exploring the Five Paths of Yoga to Reclaim Your Expressive Spirit*
Erin Byron, MA

Combining expressive arts and yoga therapy, *Yoga for the Creative Soul* is an invaluable guide to healing emotional wounds and creating a joyous life. Through drawing, writing, dancing, humming, and cooking—as well as yoga postures, meditation, relaxation, breathing, and self-inquiry—this book helps you cultivate your true intentions and live your deepest values.

With helpful tips for daily practice and a quiz to support you in identifying areas of imbalance, author Erin Byron shares techniques that you can personalize to meet your specific needs. Discover how to bring color, movement, and melody into everyday moments with the five paths to self-realization: Karma, Jnana, Raja, Bhakti, and Tantra. Engaging a process of personal transformation and learning how take control of your life are gifts you can give yourself with *Yoga for the Creative Soul.*

**978-0-7387-5218-1, 240 pp., 6 x 9**                              **$17.99**

---

**To order, call 1-877-NEW-WRLD or visit llewellyn.com**
**Prices subject to change without notice**

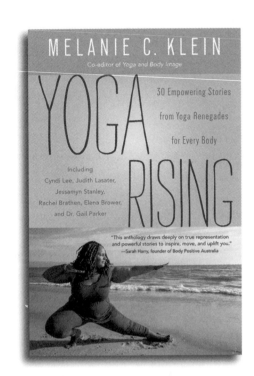

MELANIE C. KLEIN

Co-editor of Yoga and Body Image

YOGA

30 Empowering Stories

from Yoga Renegades

for Every Body

Including
Cyndi Lee, Judith Lasater,
Jessamyn Stanley,
Rachel Brathen, Elena Brower,
and Dr. Gail Parker

RISING

"This anthology draws deeply on true representation
and powerful stories to inspire, move, and uplift you."
—Sarah Harry, founder of Body Positive Australia

## Yoga Rising
### *30 Empowering Stories from Yoga Renegades for Every Body*
### Melanie C. Klein

*Yoga Rising* is a collection of personal essays meant to support your journey toward self-acceptance and self-love. This follow-up to the groundbreaking book *Yoga and Body Image* features thirty contributors who share stories of major turning points. Explore how body image and yoga intersect with race and ethnicity, sexual orientation, gender identity, dis/ability, socioeconomic status, age, and size as part and parcel of culture and society.

Collectively, we can make space for yoga that is body positive and accessible to the full range of human diversity. With a special emphasis on how you can take action to build community and challenge destructive attitudes and structures, *Yoga Rising* is a resource for the continuing work of healing ourselves and our world as we move toward liberation for all.

**978-0-7387-5082-8, 336 pp., 6 x 9**                                          **$17.99**

**To order, call 1-877-NEW-WRLD or visit llewellyn.com**
**Prices subject to change without notice**

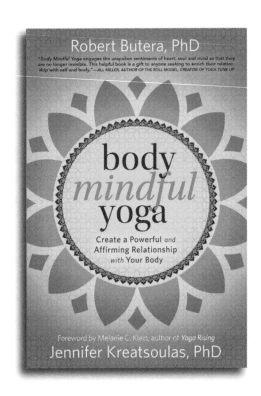

Robert Butera, PhD

"*Body Mindful Yoga* engages the unspoken sentiments of heart, soul and mind so that they are no longer invisible. This helpful book is a gift to anyone seeking to enrich their relationship with self and body."—JILL MILLER, *AUTHOR OF THE ROLL MODEL, CREATOR OF YOGA TUNE UP*

# body *mindful* yoga

Create a Powerful *and* Affirming Relationship *with* Your Body

Foreword by Melanie C. Klein, author of *Yoga Rising*

Jennifer Kreatsoulas, PhD

## Body Mindful Yoga
### *Create a Powerful and Affirming Relationship with Your Body*
#### Robert Butera, PhD, and Jennifer Kreatsoulas, PhD

Learn to transform negative words, thoughts, perspectives, and beliefs into empowering ones with *Body Mindful Yoga*'s unique approach to combining yoga and the power of language. The words you think, speak, and absorb inform how you feel about your body. With this book's inspiring guidance, you can begin to move through the world with an attitude that radiates self-confidence, contentment, and peace of mind and body.

Open your eyes to how words affect your body image using four Body Mindful steps: Listen, Learn, Love, and Live. These steps provide powerful insights, techniques, and hands-on exercises. The latter two steps encourage active practice as you improve your inner life (the words you speak to yourself) and your outer life (your interaction with others). This book shows you how to be a Body Mindful ambassador who empowers yourself and everyone around you.

**978-0-7387-5673-8, 240 pp., 6 x 9**                                        **$17.99**

---

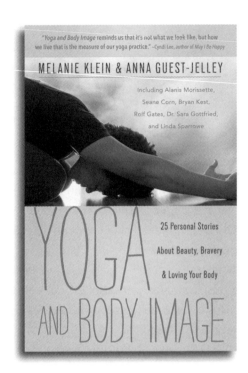

"Yoga and Body Image reminds us that it's not what we look like, but how we live that is the measure of our yoga practice." –Cyndi Lee, author of May I Be Happy

MELANIE KLEIN & ANNA GUEST-JELLEY

Including Alanis Morissette, Seane Corn, Bryan Kest, Rolf Gates, Dr. Sara Gottfried, and Linda Sparrowe

# YOGA AND BODY IMAGE

25 Personal Stories About Beauty, Bravery & Loving Your Body

# Yoga and Body Image
### *25 Personal Stories About Beauty, Bravery & Loving Your Body*
### Melanie C. Klein and Anna Guest-Jelley

In this remarkable, first-of-its-kind book, twenty-five contributors—including musician Alanis Morissette, celebrity yoga instructor Seane Corn, and *New York Times* bestselling author Dr. Sara Gottfried—discuss how yoga and body image intersect. Through inspiring personal stories you'll discover how yoga not only affects your physical health, but also how you feel about your body.

Offering unique perspectives on yoga and how it has shaped their lives, the writers provide tips for using yoga to find self-empowerment and improved body image. This anthology unites a diverse collection of voices that address topics across the spectrum of human experience, from culture and media to gender and sexuality. *Yoga and Body Image* will help you learn to connect with and love your beautiful body.

**978-0-7387-3982-3, 288 pp., 6 x9**                                    **$17.99**

---

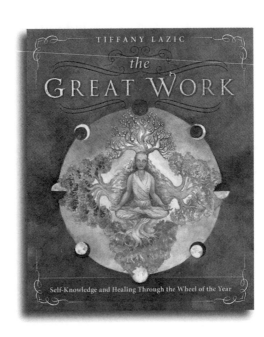

the
GREAT WORK

Self-Knowledge and Healing Through the Wheel of the Year

# The Great Work
## *Self-Knowledge and Healing Through the Wheel of the Year*
### Tiffany Lazic

Fusing ancient Western spirituality, energy work, and psychology, *The Great Work* is a practical guide to personal transformation season by season. Learn to be truly holistic by incorporating key physical, emotional, and energetic practices into your life at times when the natural tides are in harmony with your process.

*The Great Work* captures the core essence of each festival with eight key themes that span the annual cycle—a cycle that reflects human development and experience. Discover how Yule can alleviate a painful childhood, how Beltane can facilitate conscious relationships, and how Mabon can assist with determining your life's purpose. Find guidance through daily journal questions, elemental meditations, and the author's unique energy-healing technique of Hynni. With this invaluable resource for your journey of inner alchemy, you'll develop an intimate connection with the earth's impulse to create balance and harmony.

**978-0-7387-4442-1, 432 pp., 7 ½ x 9 ³⁄₁₆**                                    **$24.99**

---

**To order, call 1-877-NEW-WRLD or visit llewellyn.com**
**Prices subject to change without notice**

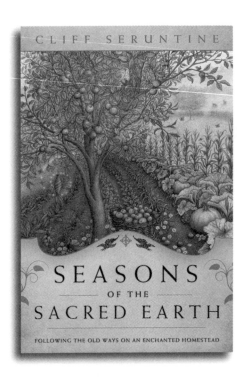

# SEASONS
## OF THE
# SACRED EARTH

FOLLOWING THE OLD WAYS ON AN ENCHANTED HOMESTEAD

# Seasons of the Sacred Earth
*Following the Old Ways on an Enchanted Homestead*
## CLIFF SERUNTINE

Join the Seruntine family on a magical journey of green living at their homestead hollow in the Nova Scotia highlands. Share their magical experiences as the family lives in harmony with the land and respects nature's spirits. Growing and hunting most of their food, Cliff and his family share hands-on practical home skills you can use, too.

With a warm, personal style, *Seasons of the Sacred Earth* chronicles the Seruntine family's adventures following the old ways. They celebrate the Wheel of the Year by leaving apples for the Apple Man, offering faerie plates during Samhain, and spilling goat's milk for the barn *bruanighe*. In return, the land blesses them with overflowing gardens, delicious ales, and the safety of their farm animals. Through their journey, you'll discover the magical and the mystical are never farther than earth and sky.

**978-0-7387-3553-5, 336 pp., 6 x 9**                              **$16.99**

To order, call 1-877-NEW-WRLD or visit llewellyn.com
Prices subject to change without notice

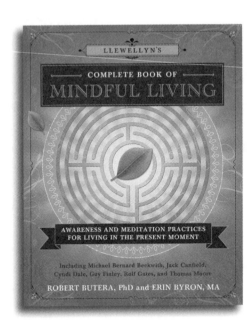

## Llewellyn's Complete Book of Mindful Living
### *Awareness & Meditation Practices*
### *for Living in the Present Moment*
### ROBERT BUTERA, PHD, AND ERIN BYRON, MA

Enhance your awareness, achieve higher focus and happiness, and improve all levels of your health with the supportive practices in this guide to mindful living. Featuring over twenty-five leading meditation and mindfulness experts, *Llewellyn's Complete Book of Mindful Living* shows you how to boost your well-being and overcome obstacles.

With an impressive array of topics by visionary teachers and authors, this comprehensive book provides inspiration, discussion, and specific techniques based on the transformative applications of mindfulness: basic understanding and practices, better health, loving your body, reaching your potential, and connecting to subtle energy and spirit. Using meditation, breathwork, and other powerful exercises, you'll bring the many benefits of mindfulness into your everyday life.

978-0-7387-4677-7, 384 pp., 8 x 10                                   $27.99

# NATURE
## SPIRITUALITY
### from the ground up

Connect with
Totems in Your
Ecosystem

LUPA

# Nature Spirituality From the Ground Up
## *Connect with Totems in Your Ecosystem*
### Lupa

*Nature Spirituality From the Ground Up* invites you to go beyond simply exploring the symbols of nature and encourages you to bury your hands in the earth and work with the real thing. This is a book on green spirituality that makes a difference, empowering you to connect with totems as a part of your spiritual life.

Uniquely approaching totems as beings we can give to, rather than take from, Lupa shows how orienting yourself this way deepens your spiritual connection to the earth and helps you rejoin the community of nature. And while most books on totems focus on animals, *Nature Spirituality From the Ground Up* helps you work with interconnected ecosystems of totems: plants, fungi, minerals, waterways, landforms, and more.

**978-0-7387-4704-0, 288 pp., 5¼ x 8**                              **$16.99**

**To order, call 1-877-NEW-WRLD or visit llewellyn.com**
**Prices subject to change without notice**